SOMATIC EXERCISES

for

NERVOUS SYSTEM

REGULATION 101

Linette Cunley

TABLE OF CONTENTS

TABLE OF CONTENTS

INTRODUCTION

Welcome! This guide is intended to help you explore new modalities to heal physical and emotional imbalances caused by common modern conditions like chronic stress, a sedentary lifestyle, and an overreliance on technology. Somatic practices can be adapted to each person's individual needs, so approach the theories and exercises with an open mind, and see which ones work best for you.

The somatic exercises in this book present an integrated approach to health and wellness, with special attention to the neurological system. If you are just beginning to explore somatic practices and body awareness, this book will help you get started. In addition, many of the exercises include variations so that you can increase or decrease the difficulty, as desired.

THE BOOK IS COMPRISED OF THREE PARTS:

Part I: **Foundations of Somatic Practice** includes an overview of the fundamental concepts and principles of somatic exercise.

Part II: **Practice** includes illustrated instructions and modifications for fifty-five somatic exercises, as well as meditations and affirmations to support health and wellness.

Part III: **28-day Somatic Evolution Plan** will inspire you to organize your practice and track your progress.

EXPECTATIONS

If you practice with consistency and heart, these exercises will help you know yourself more deeply, and appreciate the wisdom of your body. These exercises do not have to be practiced alone. If you can practice with others, you might find that you practice more consistently, help each other perform the exercises correctly, and achieve more results than you might achieve alone.

PRECAUTIONS

It is important to clarify that no matter how simple the exercises might seem, it can be helpful to consult with a specialist before beginning, especially if you have experienced severe trauma, injury, or serious health problems. Therapeutic support from a therapist trained in somatic practices can be especially helpful if you notice any strong emotional responses when performing the exercises.

FOUNDATIONS OF SOMATIC PRACTICE

I

"The human body is not an instrument to be used, but a realm of one's being to be experienced, explored, enriched and thereby educated."

Thomas Hanna

Somatics is the practice of exercises that benefit the mind-body connection. All of the terms are inspired by the perspective that the body, mind, and spirit can be fine-tuned to work together in harmony. Somatic interventions can include meditative exercises focused on breathing, visualization, body movement, and alignment. These develop both proprioception (awareness of your body and its movement in space) and interoception (connection with your inner feelings and sensations).

If you practice somatics regularly, you can achieve a deep, conscious, and happy connection with yourself in the here and now. Somatic practices teach you to stay physically present in the moment and not get lost in your thoughts, worries, or stress. This guide takes a holistic approach: each exercise includes information about the psycho-emotional, physiological, and structural dimensions of the exercise.

The word **soma** is usually interpreted as a synonym for "body," but it goes beyond that. Soma refers to the understanding of your organism as a living whole, through which your mind and soul express themselves. So, whenever you use the word soma, instead of focusing on the material flesh of your body, connect it with the marvelous and divine intelligence existing within it[1]. The body's intelligence allows you to synchronize intuition, intelligence, and emotional expression as you perform each exercise.

EMBODIMENT

"Embodiment means we no longer say, I had this experience; we say, I am this experience."

Sue Monk Kidd

Embodiment means fully experiencing your presence in the here and now. An embodied state represents cohesion, health, and authenticity. Therefore, developing embodiment will help you to truly be yourself, in harmony with both internal and external demands. When you practice embodiment it can allow you to contemplate your own consciousness with perceptive clarity, and find new ways to connect with a sense of well-being. This is the fundamental goal of somatic exercises; technical perfection of the exercises is not necessary. Instead, focus on deepening your awareness of the thoughts, feelings, and perceptions you experience during the practice, and then try to consciously integrate that sense of embodiment into your daily life.

Dissociation is the opposite of embodiment. Although the term is sometimes used to describe severe psychic disorders, in reality many people experience some dissociation, however mild. Dissociation is a natural consequence of traumas and unresolved psycho-emotional wounds, and it can feel like numbness, a disconnection from the body, or an inability to self-regulate[4]. Somatic exercises can help resolve feelings of dissociation so that you can more fully experience embodiment, integration, and well-being.

In **somatic therapy**, a practitioner works with a trained therapist to practice a broad range of somatic exercises and mind-body awareness to promote healing and well-being. Somatic therapy can be practiced alone, or incorporated with other therapeutics by professionals, including nurses and physicians, physical therapists, psychotherapists, osteopaths or holistic practitioners, as well as yoga, qigong, and Pilates instructors.

Somatic exercises are generally safe for everyone. However, if you are experiencing severe trauma or health conditions, psychiatric disorders, social isolation, or depression, it can be helpful to work with a somatic therapist. It can also be helpful if you are pregnant, post-partum, or if you would simply like to deepen your somatic practice and healing process.

SENSATIONS, EMOTIONS, THOUGHTS, AND SENTIMENTS

Although the following terms are frequently used, they are commonly misunderstood, or conceptualized differently than we might use them in somatics. It is valuable to briefly address them, especially to help you understand your power over them.

Sensations are everything that is received and processed through the senses, like taste, touch, smell, vision and hearing. The senses that most concern somatic practices are the inner senses, proprioception and interoception. When practicing embodiment, try to reconnect with your feelings, especially those related to the internal senses. Later in the book, we'll explore proprioception and interoception at length.

Emotions emerge as a response to what you feel both externally and internally. The five predominant emotions are: love, joy, fear, sadness, and anger. Emotions involve organic processes, but are usually connected to patterns influenced by your psyche, lifestyle habits, and situations in daily life. Therefore, when you become aware of these patterns, you can free yourself from conditioned reactivity.

Thoughts are the products of mental activity involving memory, language, sense of self, space, and time, in conjunction with what is perceived through both external and internal senses. Thoughts have a direct effect on your emotions and your response to situations. However, conscious breathing and various psychotherapeutic resources can help you learn how to regulate your thoughts in positive ways.

Sentiments are your interpretations of different emotions and sensations received through the senses. These responses—both mental and physiological in nature—extend over time and are strongly influenced by cognitive patterns and conditioning.

STRESS V. EUSTRESS

Stress can be experienced in many ways, but it often feels like a state of imbalance or disharmony. Stress responses have a clear psycho-emotional and even spiritual component and they are expressed in all dimensions of the self. However, despite its bad reputation, stress is not always negative.

Stress responses allow us to adapt to both external and internal demands in favor of survival and happiness. This manifests itself in the recovery of balance (or eustress), and yet it's important to note that balance is not static. Balance is fluctuating, and needs to be found again and again. Chronic stress is like leaving an engine on overdrive; over time, it can deplete energy reserves, and cause chronic physical and psychological imbalances[9].

BODY AND PHYSIOLOGY

Now that we have reviewed the holistic essence of the somatic approach, it is time to go into the structural and physiological elements involved in somatic practice, keeping the focus on integral and neurological health. The body integrates multiple systems that are designed to function in harmony. Together, the nervous, endocrine, and immune systems respond to stress, so if stress is poorly managed it can negatively impact the health of these systems.

THE NERVOUS SYSTEM

The nervous system transmits electrical and biochemical signals throughout the body almost instantaneously. Our ability to feel, move and think depends on the nervous system, which is divided into two main parts: the central system and the peripheral system[10]. Somatic exercises focus on the central nervous system, starting with the brain. Somatic exercises that emphasize conscious breathwork, focus, and body movements can lead to better brain performance, and influence your capacity for thought, language, memory and emotional control, as well as the regulation of biorhythms and mental activity in general.

Likewise, somatic stretches that increase back flexibility can improve the transmission of nerve impulses in the spine and the peripheral nervous system[10] and support optimal functioning in the organs, glands and viscera. In addition, maintaining proper hydration improves the flow of cerebrospinal fluid[11], which is responsible for nourishing, protecting, cleaning and lubricating the spinal cord, and can prevent nerve damage and improve vitality.

The peripheral nervous system is composed of the other nerve cells outside the central nervous system, which transmit nerve impulses between the central nervous system and the periphery of the body (muscles, senses, organs and viscera). The **vagus nerve** originates from the medulla oblongata in the brain stem, and has a direct relationship with the regulation of stress and a large part of the physiological processes. This is reflected in its innervations to the heart, bronchi, liver, pancreas, stomach, larynx, pharynx, spleen, kidneys, intestines, and ear.

The voluntary nervous system is linked to all the actions we perform at will, especially with respect to movement. And, the autonomic or involuntary nervous system, which is the one that without our direct control (although we can influence it) regulates a great part of our physiology[10] including heart rate, breathing rate, body temperature, digestion, sexual arousal, pupillary response, and excretion. This system can benefit from somatic practice, and it has a direct relationship with our ability to regulate stress[8].

The sympathetic nervous system is in charge of fight-or-flight stress responses and is related to the activation of energy-consuming processes[8] like metabolism to release the energy we need in times of stress. When chronic stress sets in, the body's resources can become depleted.

The parasympathetic nervous system is responsible for activating digestion, states of calm and energy reserve, and anabolic and tissue repair processes. It plays a leading role during sleep and stress management.

The enteric nervous system plays a crucial role in mood regulation and intestinal motility. It is strongly influenced by nutrition, stress, and physical activity.

The inner senses (interoception and proprioception) are not as well known as the other senses (hearing, smell, taste, touch and sight), but they have a fundamental role in somatic practice because they are essential for the processes of insight and body awareness. **Interoception** is the sensitivity to stimuli generated within the body. **Proprioception** is the sensitivity to the body's orientation in time and space. Together, interoception and proprioception allow you to deeply feel embodiment from the inside out.

THE ENDOCRINE SYSTEM

The endocrine system and main glands secrete hormones into the body and their functioning has a direct effect on emotional regulation and stress response. The main endocrine glands include: the adrenals, gonads, pancreas, liver, thymus, thyroid, and hypothalamus-pituitary axis.

The adrenals secrete hormones directly related to stress responses: adrenaline, noradrenaline and cortisol[15]. On an emotional level, their imbalance is associated with the accumulation of fears and guilt. Exercises that stretch and flex the middle and lower back help regulate them.

The gonads (testicles and ovaries) secrete hormones responsible for the regulation of reproductive functions and sexual arousal[15]. Their imbalance is associated with sexual trauma and the loss of inspiration and creativity. In somatics, we regulate its activity with pelvic floor and sphincter contractions.

The pancreas secretes hormones related to metabolism and digestion[15]. Its imbalance is associated with problems with honor and self-acceptance.

The liver is an organ that fulfills many functions like the secretion of hormones that regulate blood glucose, metabolism and regulation of the endocrine system[16]. Its imbalance is associated with accumulated anger, loss of initiative and frustration. It is regulated somatically together with the pancreas by practicing dynamic breathing exercises.

The thymus helps the maturation of immune cells[17]. Its imbalance is associated with resentment and lack of maturity in love and compassion. It is worked through gentle tapping or cupping on the area between the lungs and behind the sternum.

The thyroid and parathyroid glands regulate metabolism and help to synchronize physiological processes[15]. An imbalance is associated with communication problems and not acting in accord with one's conscience. In somatics its functioning is regulated with movement to realign the head and neck, singing, and breathwork.

The hypothalamus-pituitary axis consists of glands regulating homeostasis, body temperature and appetite, as well as mating and aggressive behaviors[15]. The glands can be regulated through nutrition, aligning sleeping and eating schedules according to natural biorhythms, and conscious breathwork.

THE IMMUNE SYSTEM

The immune system is the defense system of the human body, and it responds to both physical and psycho-emotional threats. When stress isn't resolved, the immune system consumes a large part of its energy reserves as it tries to stay on the defensive, and over time this can lead to chronic health problems, including inflammation[8].

In somatic therapy, the immune system can benefit from chest opening exercises, body alignment, and massages that stimulate lymphatic drainage. At the psychotherapeutic level, it helps to forgive and release stored sadness.

PRINCIPLES OF SOMATIC EXERCISES

These exercises will help you heal, and feel better in general. They will also allow you to develop a more conscious and loving relationship with your body and soul. Somatic exercises respond to a profound paradigm about integrative health. Therefore, to understand and appreciate their benefits, it is necessary to know some principles.

FIRST PRINCIPLE: YOUR BODY IS THE TEMPLE OF YOUR SOUL

It is normal and sensible to take care of the home in which we live. We know that the appearance and order of it influences our well-being, as well as the image we project about ourselves. Now, if we feel this with our home, how can we not feel it with the body we inhabit throughout our lives? We come from an era when popular culture taught us to see the body as banal. However, somatic exercises show that the body is sacred too. It may be challenging for the ego to embrace this truth, but it is healing to love and listen to the body.

AFFIRMATIONS

- "My soul lives in every cell of my body."
- "My body is sacred and wise."

SECOND PRINCIPLE: BODY, MIND, AND SPIRIT ARE ONE

The more we accept that the body is sacred and wise, the less we can ignore that everything that happens to it (and hurts) is an expression of our mind and emotional state. We also need to recognize that we have entered an era where routines and jobs have become more sedentary. This attenuates the connection with the body and can compromise your health. Every pain, limitation, or improvement you perceive are signals to listen to. Connecting with your body also helps you to better anchor yourself to the here and now and experience embodiment.

AFFIRMATIONS

- "I live consciously in the here and now."
- "My spirit, body, and mind are in unity."

THIRD PRINCIPLE: BREATHING IS KEY

Breathing is not only about the exchange of oxygen for carbon dioxide carried out by the lungs. This is a function that involves the whole body, apart from the fact that it is not just about air, but about nutrients and energy.

Ancient traditions such as yoga and qigong have always focused on breathing correctly. It is the main bridge between body and mind, and key to effective practice[17]. For example, an indicator that you are performing an exercise correctly and safely is that you can breathe deeply without tension or discomfort.

Also, becoming aware of how you breathe will help you maintain self-control and regulate any emotional reactions[18]. However, despite its simplicity and availability, it is easy to forget. The key is to develop a practice that helps you remember to breathe in difficult moments.

AFFIRMATIONS

- "I breathe deeply into the flow of life, feeling at one with the universe."
- "My whole body is a continuous channel of energy."

FOURTH PRINCIPLE: AWARENESS ALLOWS HEALING

Health problems and physical limitations are messages from the soul. When we listen to it and open ourselves to learn from it, many things will align by themselves, almost like magic!

When we get into somatic exercises, we realize that often what the body needs is to get better at self-love. You can express that love by listening to your body and healing your emotions. Implementing healthy habits is also a crucial resource. However, as you master listening to your body, you will be able to better sense what is good for you and act accordingly.

AFFIRMATIONS

"In order to heal, I dare to become aware of what I have not wanted to see."

FIFTH PRINCIPLE: YOUR BODY, YOUR TIME

True healing occurs in the here and now as you actively integrate body, mind, and spirit in the present. However, that does not mean that healing processes are immediate. Profound and lasting changes require patience and discipline, as well as time to assimilate. Remember that most health problems come out after years of imbalance and bad habits, so allow yourself time to heal as well.

It is also necessary to accept that we do not all learn at the same pace. No matter how simple an exercise may seem, if it causes you complications or if you need to go more slowly, accept it without shame. You can also switch to easier exercises or consider simpler variations.

AFFIRMATIONS

- "I accept this time to heal and grow."
- "The key is to live in the here and now with better and better fulfillment."

SIXTH PRINCIPLE: NUMBNESS, FLOODING, AND FLOW

We are beings of light and energy. Even if you wish to look at it only from the most rational and physiological perspective, this is still a fact. Trauma and chronic symptoms indicate an energy blockage, and often, the splitting and 'forgetting' of some aspect of yourself.

Therefore, when you begin to heal through embodiment, it is inevitable that you will reactivate the flow of energy in the process. In some cases, you may experience a strong sensitivity which can cause 'flooding' reactions that can feel like emotional overwhelm. Somatic work like breathing and meditation can help you consciously regulate strong feelings. After the flooding, the flow of energy will stabilize and your overall health will improve from there on.

AFFIRMATIONS

- "I am a channel of energy and healing."
- "I connect with my whole self by letting energy flow in harmony."

SEVENTH PRINCIPLE: LOOK OUT FOR THE PURPOSE AND NOT JUST THE CAUSE

Understanding the psycho-emotional causes of imbalance is important. However, focusing only on what caused the imbalance can trap you in rigid logic and blocked feelings. As spiritual beings, we have the opportunity to learn new things, expand our consciousness, promote change, and heal. Focus your attention on healing.

Some ailments and discomforts are caused by repressing our instinct to evolve and move on to new stages of life. In addition, as each soul is unique, this helps to understand that even with the same symptoms, the outcome or solution may vary from person to person. Therefore, do not close yourself off, compare yourself with others, or judge them. Embrace the uniqueness of your process.

AFFIRMATIONS

"Without prejudice, I am evolving on my soul's unique path."

BONUS CONTENT

We want to see you achieve your goals. To help, I've included bonus resources with you in mind: Easy-to-follow Video Tutorials, Printable Trackers, Illustrated Posters and more.

BONUS #1 | **Video Tutorials** - Get unlimited access to easy-to-follow video tutorials that guide you through how to do every exercise in the book.

BONUS #2 | **Printable Trackers and Illustrated Posters** - Stay motivated and track your progress with weekly printable guides.

BONUS #3 | **7-Step Guide to Kicking Fear and Anxiety** - This guide helps you build your confidence and commit to establishing a new wellness routine.

BONUS #4 | **Guided Meditations** - Immerse yourself in calming guided meditations designed to support your wellness journey.

BONUS #5 | **Facebook Community** - Connect with like-minded individuals, share your progress, ask questions, and receive ongoing support and motivation from both peers and experts.

THE LINK AND PIN CODE TO UNLOCK YOUR BONUS
IS ON THE LAST PAGE OF THIS BOOK.

These bonuses are **FREE** and designed to **help you achieve your goals**.

PRACTICE

Now it's time to practice! You have already learned much of the theory and principles necessary for a comprehensive understanding of somatic exercises, and now you are ready to begin.

HOW TO USE THE EXERCISES

This guide is designed for beginners, and introduces somatic exercises that prioritize an awareness of "beingness" as you practice. We have organized the exercises to make it easy for you to perform them in an adaptable, safe, and effective manner. Each exercise includes instructions, along with meditation suggestions and tips for modifying the poses to best suit your individual needs.

First, we will teach you some basic somatic concepts and skills to help you begin, followed by two stages:

Foundational Resources: Each somatic practice session is an encounter with yourself. Perform the exercises with awareness for a deep and enriching experience.

Stage One: Wellness for Everyone. These anti-stress and basic self-regulation exercises are designed to help you find a sense of balance in the easiest and most effective way possible. Therefore, they are more generic in application, addressing the most systematic and common problems.

Stage Two: Calibrating Body, Mind, and Spirit. The exercises in this stage can relieve many common health challenges. Let these harmony and longevity exercises inspire you to delve more deeply into specific aspects of your overall sense of health and well-being. You can also cultivate harmony and self-awareness beyond symptom relief.

THE INTRODUCTION TO EACH SET ALSO INCLUDES
THE FOLLOWING RESOURCES:

- A brief research-based explanation on the topic being addressed, how it's related to the nervous system's health, and why somatic exercises are effective for it.

- A list of the main psycho-emotional causes of imbalance and meditation prompts to help you find balance.

- Holistic lifestyle tips to support positive change.

ORGANIZING YOUR PRACTICE

The exercises in each stage are organized by the themes or problems they address. Within each set, the practices are autonomous and effective on their own. However, try using them all together for a more holistic practice.

Each set includes a simple breath practice, a series of exercises, and a restorative or integrative exercise which should take approximately fifteen to twenty minutes to complete. However, you are free to use them as you like, both in order and duration. A deep somatic practice can take at least four to five minutes per exercise. You can also mix your favorite exercises from different sets in a personalized series. In the final section of the 28-day plan, you will find more ideas on how to customize an exercise routine.

TERMINOLOGY

Here are some common terms you will encounter throughout the exercises:

CHIN LOCK

This is the safest way to align the head and neck. It consists of bringing the chin back (not down, except when indicated), keeping the head upright, aligned with the spine. This lock allows an adjustment of your cervical and endocrine system, in addition to subtly helping with concentration. It is a safe practice in most cases, but consult your physician in case of injury or pain.

ENGAGE THE CORE

This refers to the contraction or "activation" of the pelvic floor muscles (sphincter and buttocks), and abdomen. It primarily functions as a safety measure for your back, and stabilizes the stress axis by its action on the adrenals. It also adjusts the digestive and metabolic system.

Make sure to practice it with an empty stomach. If you are pregnant, recovering from a recent abdominal surgery, or experience any significant pain while performing the exercise, please perform a modified version by only contracting the sphincter and glutes. Consult your physician if you have any concerns.

FOCUS ON THE TIP OF THE NOSE

This focus causes the eyes to partially close, and gaze softly at the ground. It allows you to connect with your body and your emotions, so that you are clear about your true feelings.

FOCUS ON THE FOREHEAD

This focus enhances the contemplation of your own thoughts in order to eliminate your identification with them and release your prejudices. It is not necessary to close your eyes when you do this.

USING PROPS: MEDITATION CUSHIONS, YOGA MATS, AND BLANKETS

You can perform the exercises on a comfortable surface such as a yoga mat, especially if you consider relaxing on your back at the end of your session. Or, you can also perform them directly on natural ground. Blankets, yoga blocks, and cushions can help when kneeling or lying face down, especially if you have any injuries or joint pain.

For seated practices, the correct position is for the knees to be at (or below) hip level. Otherwise, it can cause tension and limit your breathing capacity. Therefore, do not hesitate to use whatever props you need to find the correct posture.

SUGGESTIONS FOR CONCLUDING EACH EXERCISE

The essence of somatic practices is to deepen the connection with your own being: each exercise is a complete learning and healing experience. Therefore, at the closing of each exercise, take a couple of deep breaths, hold the air in for a few seconds, and exhale softly. Then, spend a few moments in silence to "seal" the practice and internalize the experience.

FOUNDATIONAL RESOURCES

SPACE AND TIME

As much as somatic practices are about connecting internally, the environment matters too. Set up a space where you feel comfortable and inspired.

In terms of time, consider establishing a set rhythm and schedule. In general, it may be more challenging at first to stick to that self-commitment. However, as time progresses, it will feel natural to continue. The most ideal times are usually in the early morning or late afternoon.

PRAYERS AND INTENTIONS

Take a few moments to decide the purpose of each session and/or to connect with your spiritual inspiration. This is a silent resource that also allows you to connect with your feelings, and thus identify a particular need for each session. You can also use it to close the practice with a blessing for the rest of the day.

CHANTS AND VOICE RELEASE

Singing has been proven to reduce stress. If you enjoy singing, or if you want to give it a try, consider something inspirational to start or end your practice. Even if you don't know how to sing, simple alternatives such as chanting or intoning vocals and feeling the resonance in your body can be very comforting. If you know how to play an instrument, you can integrate that into your practice as well.

BODY SCAN PRACTICE

This resource is a must in somatic therapy, and you can also integrate it into your personal practice. Take a few moments to visualize your body, part by part, and identify where there might be physical or emotional tenderness that could be attended to during the practice. Take time to recognize and value each part of yourself. Everything that happens in your body also happens in your mind and spirit, so your body is you.

"SHAKE IT OFF"

This is another very useful exercise to let go of stress, and be more willing to be present in the here and now. Vigorously shake your whole body for at least half a minute. If you are standing, you can jump as well as shake. You can also perform the exercise while lying down or sitting. At the end, inhale deeply, stretch your body and arms up as much as possible, and then tighten all of the muscles in your body, then exhale and relax to release the tension.

DANCE

Whether with music or in silence, dance can be a fun and creative way to establish connection with every part of the body. To do this, make sure that when you are done, all the muscles have moved. Integrating music and movement will activate your sense of alertness to the here and now.

When you finish, spend a few seconds in silence. Chances are you will feel your heartbeat clearly, which will create a more intimate inward connection during the practice.

PROGRESSIVE DIAPHRAGMATIC BREATHING

Correct breathing is essential in any effective somatic practice. Recognizing and training diaphragmatic breathing before your session will help to maintain it more naturally during the exercises and clear your mind.

Begin by placing your hands on your belly. As you inhale, feel the diaphragm expand downward, massaging the organs and viscera in the abdomen. It is even more ideal that you do this while simultaneously contracting the pelvic floor, without expanding the belly. When exhaling, be sure to release all of the air.

TIPS

- If it causes you to yawn, it means that the diaphragm is 'asking' you to breathe even deeper, so that the lateral ends of the diaphragm also move.

- If you wish, you can deepen this practice by trying to breathe more deeply and slowly with each cycle.

- You can also incorporate breathing into body scanning: inhale and visualize the air moving through each part of your body. Become aware of any tension and pain you find along the way. Imagine that this pure air, like a gentle breeze, brings peace and healing to every corner.

- Although it is suggested for the introduction of a practice, you can also use diaphragmatic breathing as a form of meditation at the end of a session.

SAVASANA (OR "CORPSE POSE")

This pose traditionally closes a yoga class. It consists of lying on your back on the yoga mat, with legs and arms comfortably stretched out and relaxed on the floor. This completely horizontal posture is ideal for closing any practice, as it equalizes and balances.

It is important to note that, for this posture, you have to lie down and apply a chin lock without a pillow, unless you have a spinal problem that requires it. A minimum of five minutes is recommended.

RELAXING EAR MASSAGE

One of the extensions of the vagus nerve reaches the ears, so its stimulation has a direct action on vagal tone regulation. The massage needs to be very soft, pressing slowly along the whole extension of the ear. Imagine that the pressure applied barely reaches the most superficial layer of the skin, sometimes becoming more of a caress than a massage.

This is an ideal exercise to practice at the end of a set, after performing other more dynamic exercises or breathwork. It is contraindicated in the case of low blood pressure.

HEART RATE VARIABILITY MONITORING

Modern technology offers wonderful tools for managing stress and overall health, even without the need for symptoms. One of these very accessible resources are mobile applications and devices for measuring heart rate variability (HRV), which is a very accurate indicator of psychophysiological health. You can use a HRV monitor to quantify the effects of your somatic and meditative practices. Consider using this technology to keep track of your evolution, especially in case of trauma or chronic health conditions. You can also use it before and after each session to evaluate the effect of specific practices.

JOURNALING

It can be valuable to keep a record of your experiences during your somatic practices. Although the most essential things are always captured in your memory and health, writing them down will help you to process and integrate the experiences. It is also an excellent resource to identify ways to deepen your practice as it evolves over time.

YOU CAN USE THE JOURNAL IN ONE OR MORE OF THE FOLLOWING WAYS:

- As an intimate record of the somatic experiences.

- As a record of symptoms and behaviors relevant to your situation or health problems you are attending to. For instance, in case of sleep problems, recording your bedtime and wake-up times, as well as notes about your day-to-day energy and sense of well-being.

- As a place to document your HRV and other vital signs to monitor your evolution.

STAGE ONE: WELLNESS FOR EVERYONE

Set I: Self-Regulation, Calmness, and Rest

"Worrying is carrying tomorrow's load with today's strength—carrying two days at once. It is moving into tomorrow ahead of time. Worrying doesn't empty tomorrow of its sorrow, it empties today of its strength."

Corrie Ten Boom

COUNTERACTING STRESS, ANXIETY, AND TRAUMA

There are many causes of psycho-emotional imbalance, including acute stress from illness, grief, divorce, life changes, financial difficulties, or an overwhelming amount of responsibilities. If you are suffering from interpersonal conflict or a lack of self-knowledge or self-confidence, that can lead to imbalances too. Somatic practices can counteract these imbalances by increasing your awareness of the present moment and reestablishing a much needed sense of well-being.

Conscious physical activity can help to regulate vagal tone and teach you to become aware of ways to moderate stress and anxiety. The aim is to use breathing and movement exercises to balance the autonomic nervous system, and foster a sense of relaxation.

When the parasympathetic nervous system is activated, you can lower energy consumption, repair tissues, improve digestion, and optimize organ function.

Finally, although all the resources in this guide can help you to learn how to heal trauma, consider doing them with the guidance and supervision of a qualified professional.

BENEFITS

This guide introduces you to somatic exercises for beginners, which will help you improve your ability to self-regulate, establish mental calmness, gain insight, and rest more deeply. You can also use the exercises to manage feelings of depression, agitation, stress headaches, and tension. The tools can be used to cope with stressful situations and panic attacks, reduce reactivity and vulnerability to stress, reduce oxidative stress levels, and regulate metabolism and vagal tone.

TIPS FOR A HEALTHY LIFESTYLE

- Try cold water therapy for quick relief: place your hands or face in cold water for two minutes.

- Actively work to improve your diet, sleep hygiene, and physical activity.

- Increase your exposure to nature.
- Regulate your use of mobile devices.
- Attend psychotherapy.
- Develop your emotional intelligence.
- Practice meditation.

SELF-REGULATION, CALMNESS, AND REST

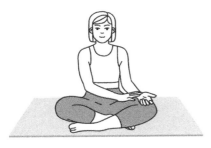

MINDFUL PULSE PALPATION

3 - 5 MINUTES

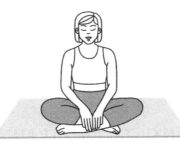

COOLING BREATH

5 MINUTES

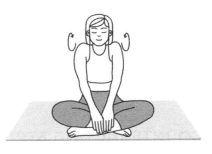

SHOULDER ROLLS

REPEAT TEN TIMES IN EACH DIRECTION

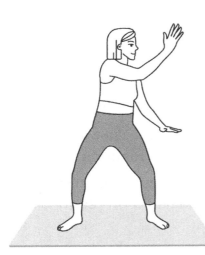

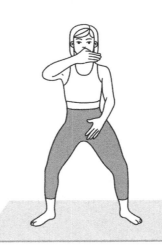

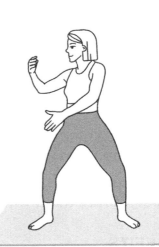

CLOUD HANDS

REPEAT 12 TIMES IN EACH DIRECTION.

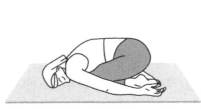

BABY POSE

2 - 3 MINUTES

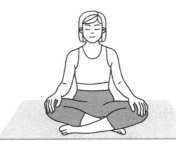

OCEANIC BREATHING

3 - 5 MINUTES

EXERCISE 1: MINDFUL PULSE PALPATION

In the womb, we listened to our mother's heartbeat. Even now, if you feel your own heartbeat, it will trigger a natural relaxation response. Use this simple and effective shortcut to regain your center.

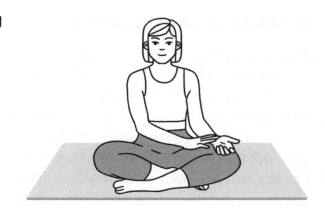

Suggested time: 3-5 minutes.

INSTRUCTIONS

1. Sit comfortably with your chest gently lifted and open. Roll your shoulders back and down. Let your eyes focus on the tip of your nose. Rest your left arm on your knee with your hand facing up.

2. Using the tips of your index, middle, and ring finger, palpate your pulse on the inner side of your left wrist.

3. Breathe deeply while paying attention to your pulse.

4. Let your consciousness merge with your heartbeat, and feel the deep peace it inspires.

TIPS

If your pulse is weak or if you find it difficult to keep your attention on it, palpate the front left side of your neck to find your carotid pulse. You can silently repeat one or two words that inspire love or calmness as you inhale and exhale.

MEDITATION

This is a very intimate meditation. It is the perfect practice to reflect on what is keeping you from yourself and causing anxiety. Use it to find answers from your soul and regain confidence.

APPLICATIONS

- Self-love and emotional awareness
- Holistic balance
- Mindful focus

EXERCISE 2: COOLING BREATH

This is a simple but very effective breathing technique that works for multiple purposes, including calming anxiety and stress. Its cooling effect is literal, because when performed correctly, you will feel a refreshing sensation. This breath slows down your metabolism, lowers blood pressure, and calms anger.

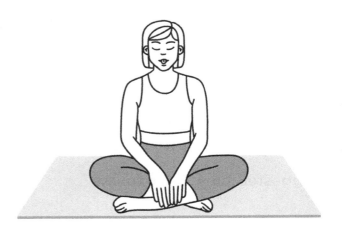

Suggested time: 5 minutes.

INSTRUCTIONS

1. Sit comfortably with your chest gently open. Apply chin lock. Focus your gaze up toward your forehead.

2. Fold your tongue into a U-shape (if you can't do this, read the variation below).

3. Inhale slowly, as if you are sipping air from a straw. Feel the cool air enter your throat.

4. Close your mouth and exhale slowly through your nose.

5. Pause for a moment at the end of the exhale, and then repeat.

TIPS

If you can't bend the tongue as required, then form a small "O" with your lips and inhale.

PRECAUTIONS

- Practice it with an empty stomach.
- Do not practice it during winter.
- Contraindications: low blood pressure; slow metabolism; obesity.

MEDITATION

Live your life calmly and patiently. This breath will evoke a more contemplative awareness, to help you live in the here and now.

APPLICATIONS

- Sleep, rest, and vitality
- Neuroendocrine and metabolic regulation
- Mindful focus

EXERCISE 3: SHOULDER ROLLS

This well-known movement can be very effective against stress. On an emotional level, the health of the shoulders is associated with the load of responsibilities and commitments we carry in life. Even if you don't have pain in this area, it is an excellent way to clear your mind and help you sleep better.

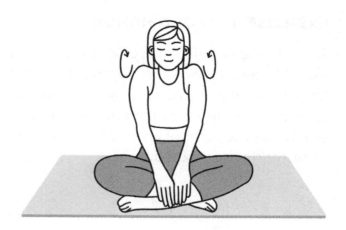

INSTRUCTIONS

1. Sit comfortably or stand up with arms relaxed, and close your eyes.

2. Begin slowly rotating both shoulders backwards. Inhale as they move up the front of the body, and exhale as they lower behind.

3. Repeat ten times in each direction.

TIPS

Variation 1: Move the shoulders vertically. Inhale as they go up, and exhale as they go down.

Variation 2: Inhale and bring both shoulders together. Hold that position with the air in, clench your fists, and squeeze all your muscles as much as possible for at least five seconds. Feel the tension in your whole body, and then exhale powerfully through your mouth, and release all of the tension.

PRECAUTIONS

Contraindications: neck or shoulder injury; migraine.

MEDITATION

Leave your problems behind; you deserve to rest. Recognize that you don't need to burden yourself to be a good person. Meditate on your commitment to follow your heart and be yourself. If you suffer from shoulder pain, consider delegating responsibilities.

APPLICATIONS

- Sleep, rest, and vitality
- Self-love and emotional awareness

EXERCISE 4: CLOUD HANDS

This classic qigong exercise is gentle, relaxing, and ideal for reminding you to take life easy. From the perspective of traditional Chinese medicine, it calms "the fire of the mind." It also lowers blood pressure and increases your respiratory capacity. Its greatest benefit is found when you perform it very slowly, and when the movement of the torso starts from the hip, gradually contracting the abdomen while exhaling.

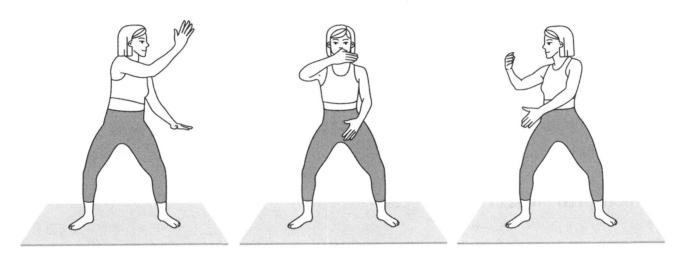

INSTRUCTIONS

1. Stand with your feet hip-width apart.

2. Turn your torso to the right. Inhale as you lift the left hand open and close to your face. The right hand stays at the height of your hips, with the palm facing down.

3. Exhale as you move your torso slowly to the left. The arms keep steady following the movement made by the torso. Keep your eyes focused on the left palm in front of you.

4. Inhale as you switch the position of your hands. Repeat 12 times in each direction.

TIPS

Keep elbows relaxed. This is a very fluid movement. As with any qigong movement, the slower the better. Focus your eyes on the tip of the little finger (this helps you calm the heart, according to traditional Chinese medicine).

MEDITATION

Let worries drift away like clouds in the sky. This movement represents the yin and yang, the eternal balance of opposites. Imagine that one hand is the sun and the other is the moon living within you, in perpetual and perfect equilibrium.

APPLICATIONS

- Holistic balance
- Mindful focus
- Spinal health and flexibility

EXERCISE 5: BABY POSE

Sometimes what we need most is to rest within ourselves. Like the previous meditation, this fetal posture evokes deep memories associated with our time in the womb and facilitates relaxation.

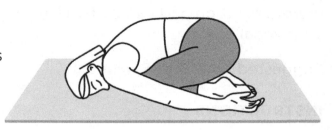

Placing your forehead in contact with the ground (or as close as possible) represents consciously making a connection with Mother Earth to let go of worries.

Suggested time: 2 to 3 minutes.

TOOLS

A yoga mat or comfortable surface, zafu, cushion, bolster, yoga block, and/or blankets.

INSTRUCTIONS

1. Sit back on your heels on your yoga mat, knees together or hip-width apart.
2. Bend your torso until your forehead touches the floor, without tensing the back.
3. Relax your arms alongside the body with palms up.
4. Keep breathing deeply, pressing your thighs with the belly on the inhale.

TIPS

Focus on the middle of your back and shoulder blades. If you feel discomfort in your legs, place a rolled towel or cushion between your glutes and heels, under your feet, or under the knees. If you feel pain in your back, try placing a cushion between your forehead and the floor. If you need something bigger, you can place the bolster between your knees and rest your torso on it, with your head turned to one side. When you bend forward, if your glutes feel tight and cannot rest comfortably on your heels, use a cushion under your forehead.

PRECAUTIONS

Contraindications: recent or chronic injury to the knees; low blood pressure; migraine, dizziness.

MEDITATION

Visualize yourself as a baby with no worries. Remember that the Earth sustains you.

APPLICATIONS

- Sleep, rest, and vitality
- Spinal health and flexibility
- Pleasure, joy, and sexual health

EXERCISE 6: OCEANIC BREATHING

This is a very soothing breath exercise that slows your breathing rate, increases your respiratory capacity, and oxygenates your blood. It also has a direct effect on thyroid function and can be healing for your vocal cords.

Suggested time: 3 to 5 minutes.

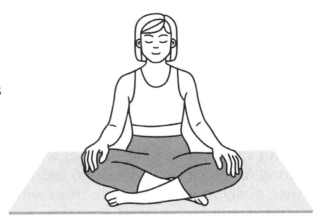

INSTRUCTIONS

1. Sit comfortably with your chest gently lifted open. Close your eyes and relax your shoulders.

2. Apply a chin lock and imagine that you are yawning with the back of your mouth and throat to lift the muscles.

3. Breathe deeply through your mouth, and briefly pause on the inhale and exhale for two to three seconds. You should hear an oceanic sound as you inhale and exhale.

4. Once you feel comfortable with it, close your mouth. Continue producing the oceanic sound as you breathe through the nose.

TIPS

Let the oceanic sound become loud. (Try to avoid a snoring sound.) If you feel any neck pain before starting, perform some neck rolls. Keep your face relaxed. The mouth breathing step is optional if you feel comfortable doing the nose breathing without it.

Variation 1: Pause on the inhalation for ten to fifteen seconds to boost its benefits.

PRECAUTIONS

*   Practice on an empty stomach.

*   Contraindications: heart problems; migraines and frequent dizziness; heart disease; pregnancy; post abdominal surgery; low blood pressure.

MEDITATION

Imagine the ocean waves purifying your body and mind. Your energy is renewed and finds balance. Such energy flows throughout your blood vessels and reaches every corner.

APPLICATIONS

*   Sleep, rest, and vitality

*   Mindful focus

*   Neuroendocrine and metabolic regulation

Set II: Sleep, Restoration, and Vitality

"True silence is the rest of the mind, and is to the spirit what sleep is to the body, nourishment and refreshment."

William Penn

The biorhythm of sleep and wakefulness is fundamental; it is the yin and yang of life. Therefore, it is crucial for a happy and healthy life to respect your needs for rest every day. Sleep allows the body to repair tissues, reduce oxidative stress, and of course, to have better energy during the day. On a neurological level, proper sleep allows for more optimal cognitive activity during the day. This improves attention and memory, as well as stress and mood management. During restful sleep, neurons are repaired, and the brain metabolizes and eliminates toxins.

Psycho-emotional imbalances can be caused by depression, worry, anxiety, guilt, or any intense emotions. You might notice a loss of rhythm and life balance, or a lack of motivation or energy. The following set offers exercises that can help you regulate your biorhythm, as well as sleep soundly and feel more energetic during the day.

BENEFITS

When you regulate the biorhythm of sleep and wakefulness, you can become aware of your power to recover your vitality, and promote a sense of peaceful consciousness. You'll also become more adept at assessing the imbalances in your general rhythm of life.

TIPS FOR A HEALTHY LIFESTYLE

- Go to sleep at a regular time (no later than 10 p.m.), and try to get seven to eight hours of sleep each night.

- Turn off lights as early as possible (including exposure to electronic screens).

- Eat dinner early so that your body has time to digest.

- Eat a light dinner with little or no carbohydrates.

- Eat more magnesium, especially from natural sources, like green vegetables.

- Moderate your consumption of coffee, chocolate, and sugar (and ideally eliminate them after 3 p.m.).

- Reduce the consumption of foods with monosodium glutamate, salt, and other flavorings that overstimulate and irritate the nervous system.

- Reduce or eliminate the consumption of gluten (wheat, barley, rye).

- Exercise regularly.

SLEEP, RESTORATION, AND VITALITY

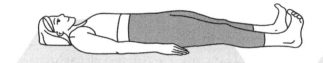
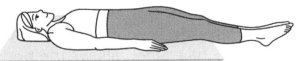

FOOT STRETCH

3 MINUTES

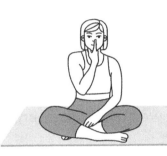

SOLAR BREATH

3 MINUTES

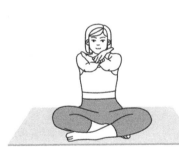
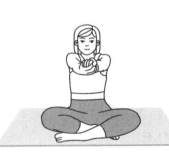

THE HEART PUMP

3 MINUTES

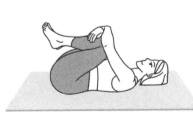

KNEE TO CHEST (APANASANA)

2 - 3 MINUTES

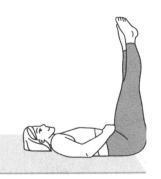

LEGS UP THE WALL

2 - 5 MINUTES

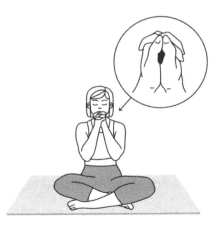

WHISTLING BREATH

REPEAT THE CYCLE FOR AS LONG AS NEEDED

EXERCISE 7: FOOT STRETCH

This simple movement, synchronized with breathing, allows you to adjust your nervous system to your body's natural needs according to the moment. If you do it when you wake up, it will help you gain mental alertness. Practicing this exercise at night does not guarantee falling asleep. However, it does help calm the mind from the day's activity.

Suggested time: 3 minutes.

TOOLS

Bed or yoga mat.

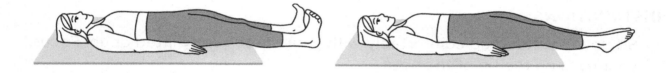

INSTRUCTIONS

1. Lay on your back without a pillow. Relax your arms and straighten your legs.
2. For relaxation: Inhale deeply as you stretch your feet, and exhale fully as you flex them.
3. For waking up: Inhale deeply as you flex your feet, and exhale as you stretch them.

TIPS

Variation 1: For a stronger effect when waking up, bring both legs together with feet stretched, and hands to your sides or under your glutes. Contract the abdomen as you raise your legs to hover in the air for three to five seconds, then release. Repeat.

MEDITATION

This exercise helps your energy flow. If you perform this exercise when waking up, imagine the energy coming out from your kidneys and adrenals and spreading throughout your body and legs.

If you perform this exercise to help you sleep, close your eyes and imagine anxiety and worries as an excess of energy stored in your head and/or upper body: visualize releasing that energy.

APPLICATIONS

- Stress, anxiety, and trauma
- Holistic balance
- Mindful focus

EXERCISE 8: SOLAR BREATH

Is it possible to start or fuel the body's engines with just one easy breathwork? Yes, it is. This handy technique stimulates the activity of the left hemisphere of the brain, which, in yogic traditions, is associated with solar polarity. It works almost immediately to give you a significant energy boost, improve focus, and stimulate digestion.

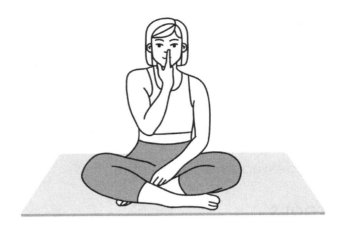

Suggested time: 3 minutes.

INSTRUCTIONS

1. Sit down or stand up comfortably with your chest gently lifted open. Focus your eyes on the tip of the nose.
2. Block your left nostril with the fingers of one hand. The other hand is relaxed.
3. Inhale and exhale through the right nostril only. Breathe deeply at a moderate pace (max. 8 seconds per cycle).

TIPS

Variation 1: Block the right nostril to inhale through the left one. Then block the left nostril to exhale through the right one.

Variation 2: Inhale fast, hold the air in for a moment, and exhale normally.

PRECAUTIONS

- Practice on an empty stomach.
- Contraindications: Pregnancy; high heart rate or blood pressure; fast metabolism; if you feel flushed, feverish, light-headed, or thirsty.

MEDITATION

Feel the sun's energy fill your body. Focus on your solar plexus and imagine that fire spreading its energy throughout the body.

APPLICATIONS

- Mindful focus
- Neuroendocrine and metabolic regulation

EXERCISE 9: THE HEART PUMP

This exercise combines a simple arm movement with powerful breathing, which will help you regain energy and enthusiasm. It is a special resource because it activates the heart while remaining in a seated position without major physical efforts. It can be a little demanding on the shoulders, so do it at a pace that feels comfortable.

Suggested time: 1 to 2 minutes.

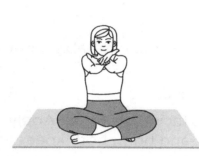 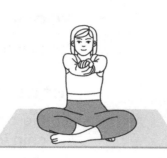 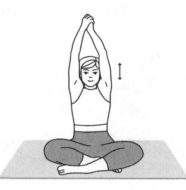

INSTRUCTIONS

1. Stretch both arms in front of you at shoulder height.

2. Bring hands together with palms facing the sky. The left hand lies on the right one. Close both hands so that the right hand grabs the left hand firmly.

3. Inhale through the nose, and move both arms up to 90 degrees.

4. Exhale through the nose, and bring your arms back down to starting position at shoulder height. Perform this exercise dynamically, with a continuous hammer-like movement.

TIPS

Your breath should be powerful and loud. Do not let the arms go lower than shoulder height. If you find it difficult to move them up to the complete vertical position, do as much as you can. Due to the strong nasal exhalation, this can help clear congestion; consider keeping a handkerchief nearby.

PRECAUTIONS

- Practice on an empty stomach.
- Contraindications: pregnancy; high heart rate; heart problems; shoulder, back, and neck injuries.

MEDITATION

Imagine lighting a fire in your heart, and raising your energy and willpower to do what you really want to do. After completing the exercise, rest, listen to your heartbeat, and connect with your soul.

APPLICATIONS

- Pleasure, joy, and sexual health
- Stress, anxiety, and trauma

EXERCISE 10: KNEE TO CHEST (*APANASANA*)

This exercise puts your mind and heart to rest (even from emotional turmoil). Knees to chest—known in yoga as *Apanasana*—is a simple, intimate, and very effective posture to calm your heart. It brings you into a fetal posture, so you can hug yourself. It is also a very effective posture to reduce menstrual pain, stretch the lower spine, facilitate intestinal motility, and optimize digestion after eating.

Suggested Time: 2-3 minutes.

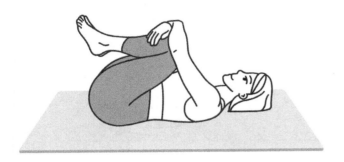

TIPS

Feel your breath as a counter-force to your legs. If you can't bring your thighs to your abdomen, then it may be more comfortable to grab your legs at the back of the knees.

Variation 1: Bring your chin closer to your neck, raising your head. Make sure you don't strain.

Variation 2: Create a pendulum motioning by bringing your chin closer to your neck, raising your head, rocking back and forth in a relaxed way for a gentle massage to your back. Keep your neck relaxed with a chin lock.

Variation 3: Perform a half Apanasana pose by hugging one knee to the chest, while the other remains straight on the floor. Hold the position for a few moments and then change.

Variation 4: To perform a core strengthening and energy release, take half Apanasana pose, then raise and lower the extended leg.

TOOLS

Yoga mat, bed, or comfortable surface.

INSTRUCTIONS

1. Lie down facing upwards. Apply chin lock and bring both knees to your chest or as close as you can and hug them together.

2. Breathe fully in the posture, while closing your eyes and relaxing.

PRECAUTIONS

Contraindications: Neck, spine, hips, or knee injury; pregnancy after the third month; during recovery from abdominal surgery; hernia.

MEDITATION

Use this posture as a reminder of the love and emotional containment you deserve. If using the posture to improve digestion after a meal, imagine food being transformed into valuable nutrients and good energy for a happier and healthier life.

APPLICATIONS

- Neuroendocrine and metabolic regulation
- Spinal health and flexibility
- Self-love and emotional awareness

EXERCISE 11: LEGS UP THE WALL

This exercise is especially for those who suffer from varicose veins and circulation problems, or who are tired from long hours on their feet. It is a good exercise to practice at the end of the day. It stimulates circulation and promotes relaxation. If you do it without resting your legs on the wall, you will also adjust the sciatic nerve and strengthen the abdomen.

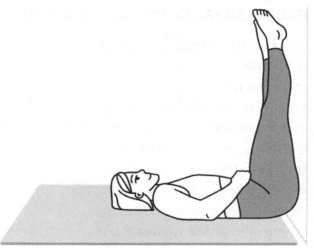

Suggested time: 2 to 5 minutes.

TOOLS

Yoga mat, bed, or comfortable surface to lie on, and a wall.

INSTRUCTIONS

1. Lie down so that your buttocks make contact with the wall or very close to it (although if you have limited flexibility, you may need to move back from the wall a little). Apply a chin lock.

2. Lift and place both legs together—and as straight as you can—in contact on the wall. Breathe deeply into the pose. If you can't stretch your legs completely from the beginning, try to do it a little more with each breath.

3. When you finish, lower both legs to the side and sit up.

PRECAUTIONS

Contraindications: Severe circulation problems; kidney problems; glaucoma; hypertension.

TIPS

Variation 1: Perform a hip opening and abductor stretch by extending your stretched legs into a wide (120-degree) angle. .

Variation 2: For core strengthening and lumbar health, perform the exercise without the wall. Keep your legs up at a 90-degree angle. Keep your abdomen contracted, so that the lumbar spine makes contact with the floor.

MEDITATION

Let go of the day's problems. Meditate on the responsibilities in your life that might be blocking your connection with yourself and your deeper feelings.

APPLICATIONS

- Spinal health and flexibility
- Grounding and sciatic nerve health

EXERCISE 12: WHISTLING BREATH

Deep and conscious breaths generally have a great capacity to relax us. However, there are some that can generate an even greater pampering effect. Exhalation stimulates rest, so this breathing is based on a very slow but deep exhalation. At the same time, the way of exhaling will generate a sound that induces a feeling of sleepiness, even in the middle of the day.

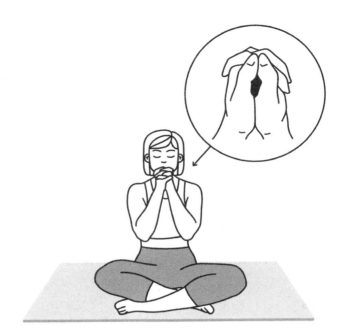

INSTRUCTIONS

1. Sit or lie down in a comfortable position.

2. Interlace the fingers of your hands at neck height (with elbows relaxed to the side).

3. Inhale normally through the nose.

4. Open your mouth like a small "o" and exhale very slowly to produce a soft whispering sound. Aim the air you exhale at the gap between your thumbs.

5. Repeat the cycle for as long as needed.

TIPS

Let your eyes gradually close. Make sure you release all the air in every exhale, so that when you inhale, the air will be automatically and powerfully pulled into your lungs.

PRECAUTIONS

Do not practice this if you are about to drive, study, work, or perform any activity that requires attention, or if you are experiencing low blood pressure.

MEDITATION

Close your eyes and let the whistling sound take over your consciousness, like a gentle breeze whispering that all is well.

APPLICATIONS

*   Stress and anxiety
*   Vagus nerve regulation

SET III. GROUNDING AND SCIATIC NERVE HEALTH

"It is only by grounding our awareness in the living sensation of our bodies that the 'I Am,' our real presence, can awaken."

G. I. Gurdjieff

Sciatica is becoming more and more frequent, mainly due to sedentary lifestyles. Our body was designed to keep moving and be in contact with nature. Therefore, abandoning both habits tends to have repercussions on our health.

Psycho-emotional imbalance can be caused by chronic stress, conflicts with home or work life, a lack of satisfying activities, or a fear of connecting with reality.

Exercises for sciatica and lower back health allow you to relieve pain in these systems, as well as vitality, and generally benefit the intestinal and reproductive systems.

In the case of grounding (standing and walking barefoot on the ground), there is increasing evidence of the benefits it brings to overall health. Some of the main ones are: regulating blood pressure and inflammation, and improving mood.

BENEFITS

If you practice somatic exercises for grounding and improving sciatic health, you can improve your sense of vitality, sexual enjoyment, and joy. The stretching and alignment postures will help with lower back and legs, and improve intestinal health. And the grounding exercises will foster a positive connection with nature and enhance your awareness of the here and now.

TIPS FOR A HEALTHY LIFESTYLE

- Adopt healthier sitting postures. Consider adjusting your chair or workstation to your height for a healthier posture.

- Take stretching or movement breaks for three to five minutes for every hour you are sitting.

- Reduce consumption of foods with artificial flavors and ingredients.

- Spend time in nature as often as possible. Embrace the natural world: try going barefoot, or hugging a tree.

GROUNDING AND SCIATIC NERVE HEALTH

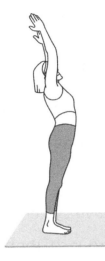

MIRACLE STRETCHING

REPEAT THE CYCLE
TEN TIMES

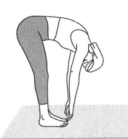

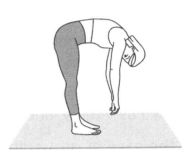

RELAXED FORWARD BEND

1 - 3 MINUTES

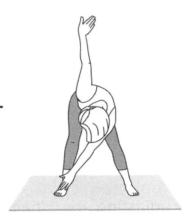

WINDMILL

1 MINUTE

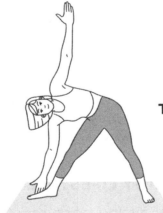

TRIANGLE POSE

1 MINUTE ON
EACH SIDE

HORSE STANCE

3 MINUTES

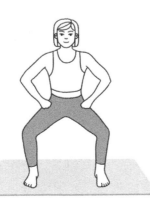

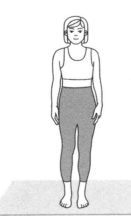

BAREFOOT WALKING

5 MINUTES

EXERCISE 13: MIRACLE STRETCHING

This is a classic stretch, but it must be performed correctly to achieve its benefits. The sciatic nerve is our cable to earth, so stretching it helps you feel firmer and increase your sense of vitality. This exercise also opens the chest and stretches the entire back. Although there is a seated version of this stretch, standing can be easier because at the end of the exhalation you get help from gravity.

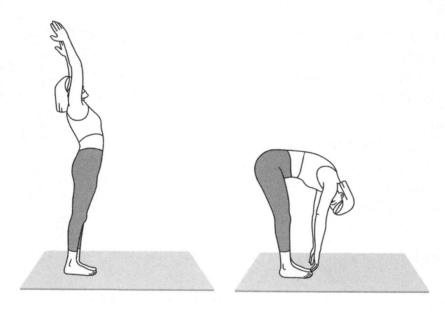

INSTRUCTIONS

1. Stand with your heels together and feet pointing out at a 45-degree angle.

2. Inhale slowly as you raise your arms above your head. Let your torso arch backward and your chest open.

3. Exhale and gently contract your abdomen as you bend your torso forward and down, reaching as low as you can. If you can, touch your feet or the floor, without bending your knees. Repeat the cycle ten times.

TIPS

To benefit the sciatic nerve, do not bend the knees. Squeeze the buttocks when reaching back (at the end of the inhalation). When you finish, stay in the final posture after you exhale; relax and breathe deeply.

PRECAUTIONS

• Practice on an empty stomach.

• Contraindications: Pregnancy, spine and neck injuries.

MEDITATION

In the open posture at the end of the inhalation, feel victorious and full of life. With an open heart, trust in yourself and the miracles you can attract into your life. As you lean forward and down, surrender to Mother Earth. Let go of any resistance, and flow with humility.

APPLICATIONS

• Spinal health and flexibility
• Pleasure, joy, and sexual health

EXERCISE 14: RELAXED FORWARD BEND

This exercise helps you to work on confidence, surrender, and relaxation. It is also very beneficial for the health of the lumbar back.

Suggested time: 1 to 3 minutes.

INSTRUCTIONS

1. From a standing position, stretch your body up on an inhale, and exhale to bring your torso forward and down.

2. Remain in the posture, without bending the knees. Let your arms fall loosely toward the floor and maintain a chin lock. Close your eyes and breathe deeply.

3. Return to standing very slowly.

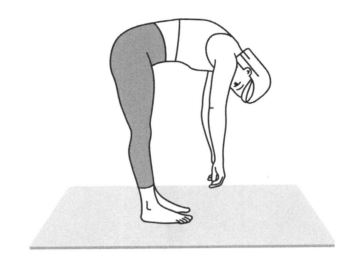

TIPS

Mentally focus your breath on your low back and feel how it relaxes as your torso releases more and more.

Variation 1: Draw circles with your shoulders (forward and backward) while your arms remain relaxed. Keep a slow and relaxing pace.

Variation 2: Let your torso make a sideways pendulum motion. Let your arms swing gently back and forth.

PRECAUTIONS

- Contraindications: Pregnancy; spine injury.

- Practice on an empty stomach.

MEDITATION

Tensions in the lower back along with sciatica are signs of not being able to trust, or be yourself. Let this posture teach you to flow with life, and regain the security of being who you are.

APPLICATIONS

- Spinal health and flexibility
- Stress, anxiety, and trauma
- Sleep, rest, and vitality

EXERCISE 15: WINDMILL

This is one of the most famous exercises for stretching the legs and sciatic nerve. It offers enough variants to adapt it to your needs and capabilities, but the main exercise is quite easy. On a mental level, it relieves stress and helps with grounding and balance. It also has an integral effect on your entire bowel system by promoting intestinal motility, and is very good for your lower back.

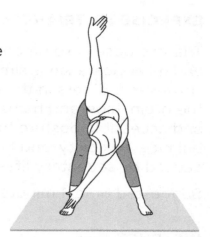

Suggested time: 1 minute.

INSTRUCTIONS

1. Stand with your feet shoulder-width apart. Your feet can point to the front or they can angle slightly outwards. Hold your arms straight and out to the sides at shoulder height. Keep your legs straight. Inhale fully.

2. Exhale and contract your navel as you slowly bring your right arm down as close as possible to your left foot without bending the knees or rolling the spine. Point the other arm to the sky.

3. Inhale as you slowly return to the starting position.

4. Exhale and repeat the movement in the opposite direction.

5. Inhale as you return again to the starting position. Continue repeating this cycle at a comfortable pace.

TIPS

Exhale fully and slowly. Let the contraction of the abdomen serve as a natural guide for downward movement. Do not roll the spine and try not to flex your knees, even if you don't go down as far as you'd like. Make sure that the overhead arm is as vertical as possible without strain. The palm faces forward to help keep your chest open and spine aligned.

Variation 1: For a bowel massage, each time you reach down, complete about three cycles of deep diaphragmatic breathing in that position before coming back up. Feel your diaphragm massaging your intestines as you breathe.

PRECAUTIONS

- Practice on an empty stomach.
- Contraindications: Hip, shoulder, spine, or neck injury; pregnancy; diarrhea.

MEDITATION

Any sciatic pain will be a message of what hurts you about the reality to which you are trying to adapt. The intestinal massage in variation 1 invites you to reflect on what toxic habits or emotions you are accumulating.

APPLICATIONS

- Spinal health and flexibility
- Holistic balance
- Neuroendocrine and metabolic regulation

EXERCISE 16: TRIANGLE POSE

Triangle pose is common in yoga practice, and its appearance is similar to the windmill. However, it differs in the fact that it also affects the groin, hips, and hamstrings. It is a relaxing and accessible posture for many. It provides balance, flexibility, and leg tension release caused by sedentary lifestyles.

Suggested time: 1 minute on each side.

INSTRUCTIONS

1. Stand with your legs positioned wider than shoulder-width apart.

2. If you start by leaning to the right side, turn the right foot so that it points out to the side at a 90-degree angle to the left.

3. Raise your arms out to the sides at shoulder height, with the palms facing down.

4. Inhale deeply. As you exhale, drop down slowly on the right side of your torso, flexing your right hip. Keep both arms straight. Try to reach as far as you can toward the right foot without bending your right knee (the left knee can have a microbend, if needed).

5. Continue to hold the position while breathing deeply. Keep facing forward with your chest open. Allow the trunk of your body to extend parallel to the floor while your hands reach in opposite directions—the right hand toward the right foot and the left hand toward the sky.

6. Slowly return to the starting position and repeat in the opposite direction. (Change the alignment of the feet accordingly).

TOOLS

Yoga block.

TIPS

Keep your legs as straight as possible. Do not rest your hand directly on your knee as this puts pressure on the joint.

Variation 1: Place a yoga block under the hand for support.

PRECAUTIONS

- Contraindications: pregnancy, neck, back, shoulder, or hips injury; migraine or headache; low or high blood pressure; diarrhea.

- Practice on an empty stomach.

MEDITATION

This posture relieves tension caused by sedentary lifestyles and fear of moving from where you are (even though you may not want to stay). Try to breathe into the challenge as you stretch in multiple directions like a star. Meditate on the sense of extending, radiating, and holding still at the same time.

APPLICATIONS

- Spinal health and flexibility
- Pleasure, joy, and sexual health
- Holistic balance

EXERCISE 17: HORSE STANCE

This exercise is good for lumbar back pain. Lumbar back health is a reflection of your connection to your instincts, livelihood, confidence, and flow with life. This exercise, known in qigong as "Ma Bu," brings awareness to this facet of your being and strengthens your roots in the earth.

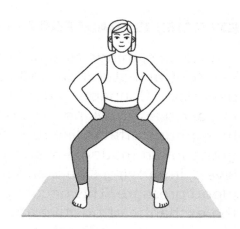

Suggested time: 3 minutes.

INSTRUCTIONS

1. Spread your legs wider than your shoulders. The wider the stance, the more difficult but effective it will be. Do not open wider than twice the width of your shoulders. Clench your fists by your hips.

2. Place your feet parallel to each other.

3. Focus your gaze on the tip of your nose, looking at the ground and absorbing its steady energy. Keep breathing deeply and visualize roots emerging from your feet.

TIPS

Practice this barefoot or on natural ground. Flex your toes so they dig a bit into the ground. Do not bring your weight to your heels; stay grounded in the front of your foot. The key to this posture is to feel the firmness and rootedness in the legs, while still staying relaxed. Take deep diaphragmatic breaths, and feel how it massages your lower back as you inhale.

Variant 1: Perform Zhang Zhuang (qigong's Tree Pose) by bringing your hands to shoulder height with your palms relaxed facing inwards, forming something very similar to a circle with the arms. Keep your elbows relaxed. Visualize that you are embracing a tree and absorbing its firmness and wisdom.

Variant 2: Perform praying pose by bringing your hands together in prayer position in front of your chest. Close your eyes and meditate on your heart getting in sync with the earth.

PRECAUTIONS

Contraindications: Ankle or knee injury.

MEDITATION

Connect intimately with the Earth. Become one with your instincts.

APPLICATIONS

- Holistic balance
- Spinal health and flexibility

EXERCISE 18: BAREFOOT WALKING

Many times, things as simple as walking barefoot on natural ground can be beneficial. Connecting directly to the earth and walking barefoot has therapeutic effects like reducing low-grade inflammation, lowering cortisol levels, improving sleep, and regulating blood pressure. This occurs thanks to the exchange of positive and negative charges between the body and the earth respectively, thus helping to restore homeostasis.

Suggested time: 5 minutes.

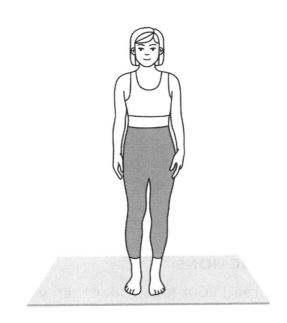

INSTRUCTIONS

1. Take your shoes and socks off.

2. Stand barefoot on natural ground and feel the earth beneath you. Close your eyes and imagine the exchange of energy between you and the earth.

3. Walk at a slow and conscious pace. Keep your feet relaxed, and feel the little twinges or tickles of the small rocks under your heels.

TIPS

Choose ground that is comfortable; very rocky soil can be uncomfortable for some people. You can also perform this exercise by sitting on a chair, or directly on the ground. If your knees come above your hips when sitting, sit on a cushion to protect your back).

MEDITATION

During barefoot walking, focus on keeping your feet relaxed. Let the rocks massage reflexology points in your feet and stimulate the nervous system.

APPLICATIONS

- Sleep, rest, and vitality
- Neuroendocrine and metabolic regulation

SET IV. SPINAL HEALTH AND FLEXIBILITY

"If you would seek health, look first to the spine."

Socrates

Science and ancient oriental traditions agree that the health and flexibility of the back is synonymous with vitality and youth. Herniated discs, tension, and pain are therefore a reflection of the wear, tear, and oxidative stress on the body. In addition, optimally functioning organs and viscera also depend on spinal flexibility and health. Low back pain, for instance, may also refer to adrenal inflammation, generally due to excessive activation of the HPA stress axis.

Psycho-emotional imbalance can contribute to problems related to mental rigidity and obsessive-compulsive tendencies; communication and pride (cervical segment); love, sociability, and self-care (thoracic segment); insecurity and livelihood problems (lumbar segment); and sex, intimacy, and personal space (sacro-coccygeal segment).

BENEFITS

Somatic exercises that focus on spinal health and flexibility will also improve posture, alignment, stability, balance, psychophysiological flexibility, and resilience to stress.

TIPS FOR A HEALTHY LIFESTYLE

- Make an effort to increase movement and physical activity.

- Practice good sleep hygiene.

- Drink half a glass of water before going to bed.

- Take care of your posture when standing for long periods of time: put your weight on the middle of your feet and not on your heels.

SPINAL HEALTH AND FLEXIBILITY

SPHINX POSE
1 - 3 MINUTES

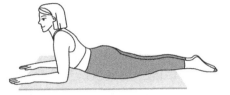

BRIDGE POSE
REPEAT TEN TIMES

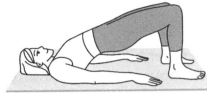

CAT-COW POSE
3 MINUTES

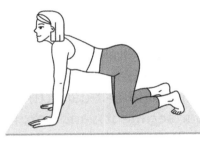
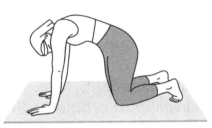

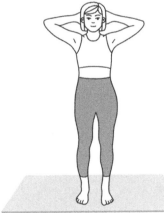
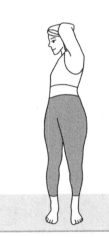

CHEST TWIST
2 - 3 MINUTES

LUMBAR BACK FLEXIONS
REPEAT THE CYCLE AT A SLOW PACE, APPROXIMATELY TWENTY TIMES

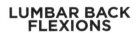
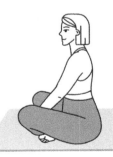
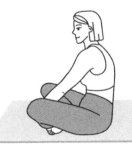

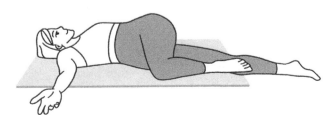

SUPINE SPINE TWIST
REPEAT THREE TIMES ON EACH SIDE

EXERCISE 19: SPHINX POSE

This is a gentle somatic exercise that works on the health and flexibility of the spine. It opens the chest, strengthens the core and adjusts the lower back. This is a perfect exercise to expand your breathing capacity and master the pelvic floor's contraction.

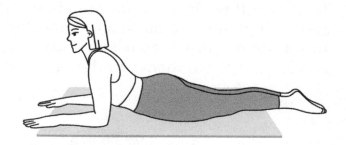

Suggested time: 1 to 3 minutes.

TOOLS

Yoga mat or comfortable surface.

INSTRUCTIONS

1. Lie on your stomach with your legs straight. Rest your forehead on the mat, your arms to the sides, and the tops of your feet on the floor.

2. Place your hands flat on the ground beside your head. With your forearms and elbows close to the torso, contract your core.

3. Inhale and feel the weight of your body on your forearms as your torso rises, and your chest opens and lifts.

4. Hold and breathe deeply for as many cycles as needed. Contract your core and glutes to keep the lower spine in contact with the mat.

5. Exhale as you lower your torso, then rest.

TIPS

Variation: Perform against a wall (during pregnancy or if having neck soreness). Stand against a wall, with arms contacting it as they would do in the sphinx pose. Mimic the sphinx's heart-opening and back-bending posture, letting your head fall slightly back and down.

PRECAUTIONS

Contraindications: Neck, back, hip, elbow, and/or wrist injury; pregnancy; headache; recent abdominal surgery.

MEDITATION

Open your heart, and with elegance and flexibility, project yourself into the future while staying grounded.

APPLICATIONS

- Grounding and sciatic nerve health
- Holistic balance

EXERCISE 20: BRIDGE POSE

This is another classic yoga pose that has many benefits. It stretches and strengthens the back, and tones the abdomen, buttocks, and legs. At a systemic level it adjusts the gonads, as well as the metabolism and endocrine system thanks to the slight pressure on the throat area (thyroid).

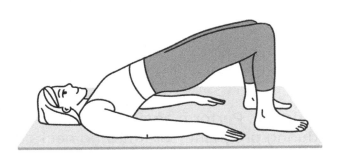

TIPS

Place a yoga block under your hips to support your weight. This variation may be needed during pregnancy. Make no force with the shoulders or arms for this exercise.

Variation 1: To decrease the challenge, grab your ankles during the exercise.

Variation 2: To increase the challenge, hold the bridge pose for a few minutes and breathe deeply.

Variation 3: For an advanced option, get into the bridge pose and, without losing the alignment, stretch one leg and foot into the air. Hold for a moment, and then return the foot to the floor. Repeat with the other leg.

APPLICATIONS

- Pleasure, joy, and sexual health
- Holistic balance
- Neuroendocrine and metabolic regulation

TOOLS

Yoga block.

INSTRUCTIONS

1. Lie on your back with your arms at your sides and palms down. Apply a chin lock. Bend your legs so that the soles of your feet rest on the floor near your buttocks.

2. Inhale as you raise your torso and thighs, until you draw a straight line from your shoulders to your knees.

3. Contract the navel and glutes and hold the lifted position for a few seconds, then exhale as you slowly return to the starting position. Repeat ten times.

PRECAUTIONS

- Contraindications: Knee, shoulder, or back injuries; severe osteoporosis.

- Practice on an empty stomach.

MEDITATION

How much are you able to elevate your basic impulses to higher intentions? The spine is the energy highway of the body, and it gives us the power to unite heaven and earth within.

EXERCISE 21: CAT-COW POSE

The cat-cow pose is a valuable and versatile exercise for the health and relaxation of the spine. It is one of the most frequently used exercises in somatic therapy, because it brings awareness and connection to the entire spine. Apart from promoting flexibility and massaging your organs, the cat-cow exercise helps to reduce stress and improve sleep.

Suggested time: 3 minutes.

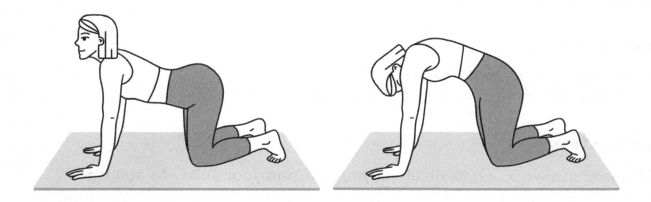

TOOLS

Yoga mat or comfortable surface, blanket or yoga block.

INSTRUCTIONS

1. Start on your hands and knees with your hands directly below your shoulders and your hips aligned with your knees to form a perfect rectangle with your body. Spread your fingers wide and straighten your spine. The tops of your feet rest on the ground and your head and neck should be relaxed.

2. Inhale as you gradually move into "cow" pose: raise your head and open your chest, with your spine curving toward the floor as your hips tilt and your stomach relaxes.

3. Exhale as you gradually move into "cat" pose: contract the navel toward the spine as your back curves upward on an exhale and your head lowers.

4. Continue moving your spine with the convex and concave curves of the cat-cow cycle for a minute or two, and then on an exhale move to child pose to relax.

TIPS

In case of neck pain, do not move your head except for what is necessary to perform the movement of the spine. Shoulders make no effort. No pain or strain should arise in them.

Variation 1: If you are pregnant, do not perform the cat pose. Focus instead on a cycle between the starting position and the cow pose.

Variation 2: Consider placing a blanket or yoga block under your knees if there is any knee discomfort.

PRECAUTIONS

- Practice on an empty stomach.
- Contraindications: Neck, spine, hip, knee, or wrist injury.

MEDITATION

This exercise works on flexibility in your life, and your ability to adapt to the here and now. Dare to overcome the conditioning that keeps you from being happy!

APPLICATIONS

- Holistic balance
- Stress, anxiety, and trauma
- Vagus nerve regulation

EXERCISE 22: CHEST TWIST

Few sensations are more pleasant than being able to breathe deeply. The more you expand your lung capacity, the greater your peace of mind and capacity to receive and give love. Chest twists facilitate opening, and in turn help the flexibility and lubrication of the middle back.

Suggested time: 2 to 3 minutes.

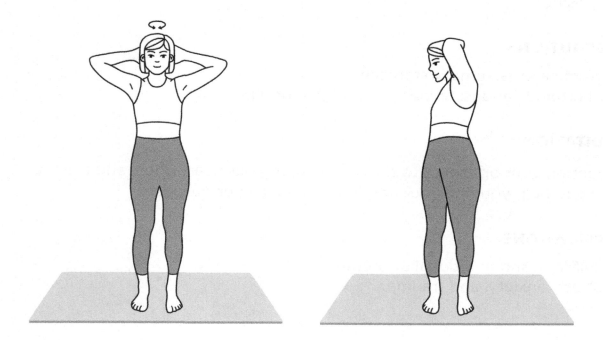

TOOLS

Zafu or cushion.

INSTRUCTIONS

1. Stand with feet shoulder-width apart. Interlace your fingers behind your neck. Open the elbows to help open the chest.

2. Inhale deeply as you rotate to the left.

3. Exhale deeply as you return to the starting position.

4. Inhale as you rotate to the right.

5. Exhale as you return to the starting position. Repeat.

TIPS

Do not let the elbows move forward. Keep the chest open. It is important to breathe fully (despite the short range of the movement) to get the desired effect. Try to make the movement fast and dynamic.

Variation 1: To open the hips, perform it in a seated cross-legged position. Make sure your legs are below your hips; sitting on a zafu can help with this position.

PRECAUTIONS

- Practice on an empty stomach.
- Contraindications: Spinal injury; high blood pressure.

MEDITATION

Reflect on your openness to the world. Keep your heart open, and trust in love to help you find your passion and fulfill your purpose.

APPLICATIONS

- Self-love and emotional awareness
- Stress, anxiety, and trauma

EXERCISE 23: LUMBAR BACK FLEXIONS

Although several of the exercises we have presented so far work on the lower back and its flexibility, this one focuses exclusively on it. These flexions are a palliative against back pain caused by a sedentary lifestyle, and help recover vitality.

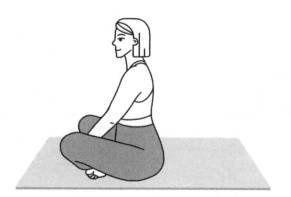 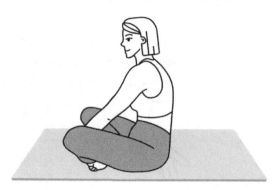

TOOLS

Chair (for chair variant).

INSTRUCTIONS

1. Sit cross-legged on the floor with both ankles in front of each other. Knees should be below the hips to prevent any strain (use the chair variation below if you can't do this). Apply a chin lock.

2. Grab your ankles firmly with both hands and keep your arms straight. The ankles won't move during the exercise, and the elbows won't bend.

3. As you inhale, open your chest as much as you can. Keep the chin lock. Your head and shoulders remain still.

4. As you exhale, contract the abdomen, so that you curl the spine, but only the lumbar segment. For this it is necessary that both the head and shoulders remain still. Repeat the cycle at a slow pace, approximately twenty times.

TIPS

If you keep your arms straight and your head and shoulders still, it will help to focus the movement on the lumbar segment. Hydrate throughout the day to help with lumbar lubrication.

Variation 1: If your flexibility is limited, sit on the edge of a chair with hands on your knees.

PRECAUTIONS

Contraindications: Spine or hip injury.

MEDITATION

How satisfying is your personal, sexual, and financial life? Is your physical activity sufficient and healthy? You can change right now and begin to make it more satisfying.

APPLICATIONS

*   Sleep, rest, and vitality
*   Grounding, sciatic nerve health
*   Pleasure, joy, and sexual health

EXERCISE 24: SUPINE SPINE TWIST

Supine spine twists are one of the best tools for ultimate back relaxation and stretching after finishing a workout session.

If done correctly, it adjusts all the segments of the back in a natural way while reducing stress and opening the chest. Use it to relieve tension and pain after sitting for a long time.

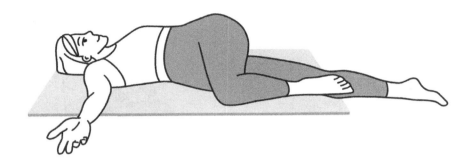

TOOLS

Yoga mat or comfortable surface, yoga block.

INSTRUCTIONS

1. Lie down on your back with your arms open to the sides and your hands facing down.

2. Inhale as you slowly bring the right leg to your chest.

3. Exhale as you lower that right leg to the opposite (left) side and turn your head to the right side. Rotate as far as you can—ideally touching the floor with your knee—but without taking your shoulders off the floor. The right foot rests on the left knee.

4. Inhale and bring back both the leg and the head to the center.

5. Exhale fully as you return to the starting position.

6. Repeat three times on each side.

TIPS

You can hold the supine twist and rest in the pose; breathe steadily and release more deeply into the twist with each breath. Once you finish, extend both arms and legs to stretch completely.

Variation 1: If you can't reach the floor with the knee, place a yoga block under the knee.

PRECAUTIONS

Contraindications: Hips, spine, knees, and neck injury.

MEDITATION

Feel that you are squeezing out the tensions and pains stored in your spine. Release any negative energy from the day to give yourself a moment of complete rest.

APPLICATIONS

- Stress, anxiety, and trauma
- Sleep, rest, and vitality
- Holistic balance

SET V. SELF-LOVE AND EMOTIONAL AWARENESS

"If your emotional abilities aren't in hand, if you don't have self-awareness, if you are not able to manage your distressing emotions, if you can't have empathy and have effective relationships, then no matter how smart you are, you are not going to get very far."

Daniel Goleman

We all have the ability to be intuitive and compassionate, and connect with our essence. However, despite this seemingly purely spiritual capacity, taking care of our body with these exercises helps to maintain and strengthen that sense. This intuition depends partly on your vagal tone, as well as knowing how to keep chronic inflammation at bay. Low grade inflammation has been shown to disrupt this capacity for introspection, causing problems with memory, concentration, and mood regulation.

One system closely linked to self-love and also chronic inflammation is the immune system, which is worn down by ongoing stress and ends up draining the body's energy. In case of autoimmune diseases, they mean that you might be living defensively or with resentment. Psycho-emotional causes of imbalance can include depression, lack of self-awareness, or unresolved trauma or bullying.

BENEFITS

Somatic practices can strengthen the immune system, alleviate depression and mood disorders, increase peace of mind, self-esteem, and your ability to express love and empathy, as well as deepen your intimacy with your body and being.

TIPS FOR A HEALTHY LIFESTYLE

- Reduce consumption of foods containing gluten, casein (dairy) and refined sugars.

- Dedicate at least 15 minutes a day for introspection and meditation.

- Take a walk in nature as often as possible.

- Attend psychotherapy.

SELF-LOVE AND EMOTIONAL AWARENESS

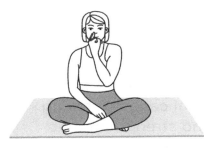

LUNAR BREATHWORK FOR EMOTIONAL AWARENESS

REPEAT TEN TIMES

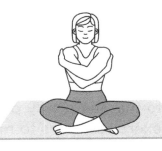

SELF-HUG

3 MINUTES

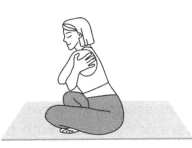

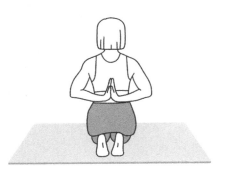

REVERSE PRAYER POSE

REPEAT FOR A FEW BREATHING CYCLES

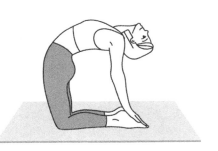

CAMEL POSE

1 - 3 MINUTES

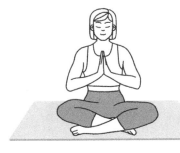

MEDITATION ON HEART PROJECTION & PROTECTION

3 MINUTES

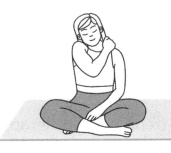

SELF-MASSAGE

3 MINUTES

EXERCISE 25: LUNAR BREATHWORK FOR EMOTIONAL AWARENESS

The moon is associated with emotions and intimacy. It also sensitively connects us with the subconscious. We have both the solar and lunar qualities in us, and when we know the right resources, we can boost them when needed.

The following breath is really simple. It can be used as an introduction to any somatic practice, in order to fine tune your ability to listen inwardly during the exercises. Lunar breathwork can awaken emotional awareness, and open ways to feel more sociable and empathetic. On an organic level, it helps you sleep and boosts both the digestion and immune systems.

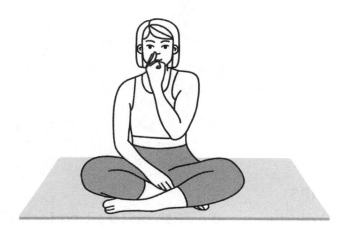

TIPS

Variation: Try alternating nostrils for a balancing effect; inhale through the left nostril, and then block the left nostril to exhale through the right one.

Go slowly: hold the air in for two seconds, and then out for two seconds.

PRECAUTIONS

Contraindicated for heart problems.

MEDITATION

Imagine a full moon illuminating your inner being. Let it relax your mind and body. Let that full moon reveal and heal the shadows of your unconscious.

INSTRUCTIONS

1. Sit comfortably with your chest gently open. Eyes focused on the tip of your nose.

2. Use the ring finger and little finger of your left hand to block your right nostril.

3. Breathe slow and deeply through the left nostril. Repeat ten times.

APPLICATIONS

- Sleep, rest, and vitality
- Neuroendocrine and metabolic regulation
- Stress, anxiety, and trauma

EXERCISE 26: SELF-HUG

One indicator of a healthy day is that you can give hugs and share lovingly with others. However, it is also comforting to hug yourself and be at peace within. This practice strengthens your breathing capacity and inspires you to love, even in hard times.

Suggested Time: 3 minutes.

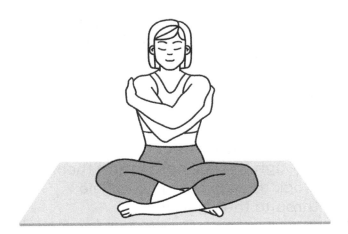 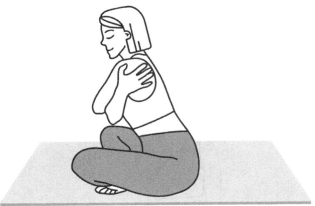

TOOLS

Chair, zafu or cushion.

INSTRUCTIONS

1. Sit either with legs crossed or on the edge of a chair. Open your chest, apply a chin lock, and close your eyes.

2. Embrace yourself so that you grab each shoulder blade with the opposite hand.

3. From this posture, tilt your body forward (about 30 degrees) with your spine straight. Breathe very deeply. Feel the counterforce produced by the embrace, and how your chest fully expands despite the pressure.

TIPS

You may need a cushion to sit on for a crossed-legged posture without strain. If it's not comfortable, try sitting on the edge of a chair.

PRECAUTIONS

Contraindications: Chest pain; arm injury; severe heart problems.

MEDITATION

Learn to love and express love even in spite of adversities. Awaken the courage in your heart to fight for love and joy.

APPLICATIONS

- Stress, anxiety, and trauma
- Pleasure, joy, and sexual health

EXERCISE 27: REVERSE PRAYER POSE

This simple posture brings your hands into a prayer position behind your back as a way to open your chest and release tension in your back and shoulders. It stretches the joints and the abdomen, and is very beneficial for your wrists. This is a practice that invites you to love even what you reject or do not yet know about yourself.

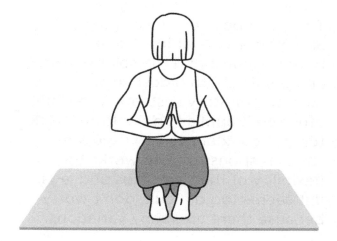

TOOLS

Cushion or chair.

INSTRUCTIONS

1. You can stand with legs shoulder-width apart, sit with legs crossed, or on the edge of a chair, whichever feels best to you. Apply a chin lock and keep your torso straight. Close your eyes.

2. Slide both arms behind your back and try to press your hands and fingertips together.

3. Breathe deeply and focus your mind on pressing into your prayerful hands as you continue to open your chest.

4. As you exhale, slowly rotate the fingertips downward to deepen the stretch and then release the posture. Repeat for a few breathing cycles.

TIPS

Variation 1: If it is difficult to press your hands together, try grabbing your elbows behind your back, opening your chest, and breathing into the stretch.

PRECAUTIONS

Contraindications: Shoulder, wrist, or back injury; low blood pressure.

MEDITATION

Recognize, love, and forgive whatever is hidden or repressed in you. Let every aspect of you find its place in your life.

APPLICATIONS

*   Spinal health and flexibility
*   Holistic balance

EXERCISE 28: CAMEL POSE

This yoga pose produces physical and mental relaxation. It opens both the chest and the solar plexus, and adjusts both digestive and cardiorespiratory systems. The slight pressure it applies on the lower back tonifies the kidneys and regulates stress response. It also works the flexibility of the back, hips and legs. If it seems too difficult, don't worry because there are many variations.

Suggested time: 1 to 3 minutes.

TOOLS

Yoga mat or comfortable surface, rolled towel, knee pad.

INSTRUCTIONS

1. Kneel on the mat with your feet flexed and your toes pressing into the floor. Apply a chin lock.

2. Inhale, and slowly lift your hips and torso up, then reach behind your body and hold onto your heels with your hands to support yourself. Contract the glutes, open the chest toward the sky, and let the spine lengthen into an arc.

3. As for the head, you can keep the chin lock, or let it drop so that you look backwards and upside down.

4. Keep breathing deeply in that posture for as long as you want.

5. To undo the posture, exhale and slowly come back to the kneeling posture.

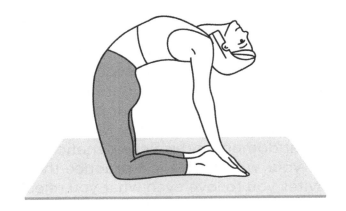

TIPS

This is a very dynamic stretch; allow your attention to stay focused on the feeling of expansion. If your neck is sore, keep the chin lock to support it. Consider using a knee pad, cushion or rolled towel under your feet and/or knees as needed.

Variation 1: If it is difficult to reach your feet, place your hands on your hips and lean your torso back as far as you can. Open the chest and lift your spine towards the sky.

PRECAUTIONS

Contraindications: Neck, back, knee injury or chronic inflammation; hernia or recent abdominal surgery; headache.

MEDITATION

You are opening your heart and pointing it to the sky. Receive infinite celestial love, and live each day with compassion. This posture may evoke a certain fear similar to vertigo. However, overcoming that feeling teaches you to love without expectations. Let go of control.

APPLICATIONS

- Spinal health and flexibility
- Sleep, rest, and vitality
- Stress, anxiety, and trauma

EXERCISE 29: MEDITATION ON HEART PROJECTION & PROTECTION

It is common to assume that your main protection comes from the physical body and tangible resources. However, your electromagnetic field has much more influence on safety and well-being than it appears. Empowering your heart and practicing self-love helps make that energetic projection more powerful and stable. In this way, you can increase your ability to be assertive, and your ability to attract others.

Suggested time: 3 minutes.

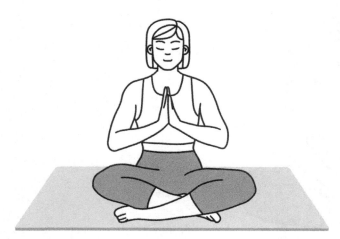 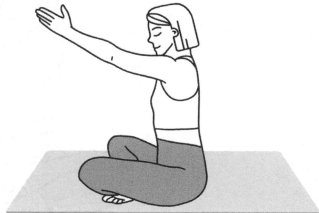

INSTRUCTIONS

1. Sit comfortably and close your eyes. Apply a chin lock. Bring your hands together in a prayer pose in front of your chest.

2. Inhale, then exhale and stretch your arms with hands still together at a 45-degree angle. Imagine that your electromagnetic field is expanded and strengthened. Any shadows or imbalance in it are cut through with your hands.

3. Inhale as you bring hands back to the starting position, like absorbing renewed energies to empower your heart.

4. Repeat the cycle.

TIPS

Mentally repeat positive and loving affirmations while performing the meditation. When you finish, stay for a few minutes in prayer posture, feeling the subtle energy of your heart.

MEDITATION

Feel your heart getting stronger and overcoming the fears that make you doubt yourself. Trust that the powers of love and spiritual peace overcome adversity.

APPLICATIONS

- Mindful focus
- Stress, anxiety, and trauma

EXERCISE 30: SELF-MASSAGE

Whether you've finished exercising or just want some self-love, massaging yourself is a nice way to connect inward. Gentle, loving stimulation of the skin helps relieve stress and ease fears. Gentle squeezing massage also stimulates circulation and detoxification.

Suggested time: 3 minutes.

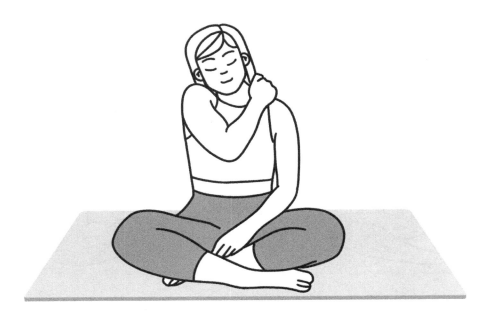

INSTRUCTIONS

Alternate caresses and massages with gentle squeezes to as many parts of the body as you can reach with your hands.

TIPS

Massage the neck, shoulders and back to help relieve tension. The jaw can accumulate a lot of anger, so focus on tenderly releasing any tension in the face and along the jawline.

MEDITATION

Love every corner of yourself. If you notice any pain as you massage, meditate on its meaning. Breathe deeply and send pure energy to that zone, and the answer will arise.

APPLICATIONS

- Stress, anxiety, and trauma
- Pleasure, joy, and sexual health

STAGE TWO: CALIBRATING BODY, MIND, AND SPIRIT

SET I. VAGUS NERVE REGULATION

"Be kind with your body–your inseparable best friend."

Manuela Mischke-Reeds

The vagus nerve plays a crucial role in the management of stress and emotions because it is the "cable" that bridges the gap between head and viscera. This stage includes a specific set of exercises and meditations for the vagus nerve, as well as exercises to help you visualize repairing and strengthening your mind-body connection. This way, you can optimize your overall health and prevent disease, in addition to healing symptoms you might be experiencing.

Psycho-emotional imbalances can be caused by common feelings of trauma, depression, guilt, shame, pride, or sexual repression. Somatic exercises that focus on healing the mind-body connection can create balance in your bio-rhythms, facilitate stress management, regulate mood, improve depression, and attune your emotional intelligence and interoception.

TIPS FOR A HEALTHY LIFESTYLE

- Follow a healthy eating schedule that pays attention to your body's natural biorhythms, with time to "rest" the digestive system between meals.

- Eat an array of whole foods that promote a healthy microbiome including fresh fruits and vegetables, fermented foods, vinaigrettes.

- Avoid inflammatory foods (with gluten, casein and refined sugar).

- Exercise regularly.

VAGUS NERVE REGULATION

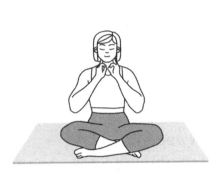

CALMING NECK MASSAGE

1 MINUTE

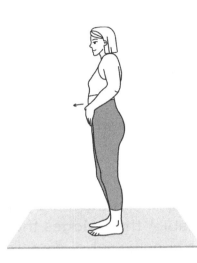
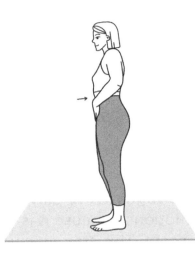

REVERSE BREATHING

3 MINUTES

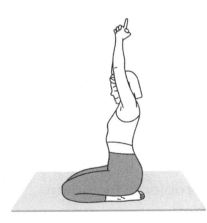

KNEELING SPINAL STRETCH

2 MINUTES

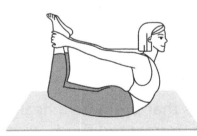

BOW POSE

STAY IN THE POSE FOR 30 SECONDS

REPEAT THREE TIMES

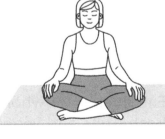

BOX BREATHING

HOLD THE AIR OUT FOR FOUR COUNTS AND REPEAT THE CYCLE EIGHT TO TEN TIMES

EXERCISE 31: CALMING NECK MASSAGE

The vagus nerve has several branches on its way down to the intestines. One of them is located in the neck, and massaging it helps to regulate vagal tone, thereby relieving stress and anxiety, among other imbalances.

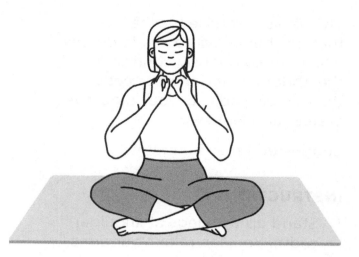

This is a simple and very accessible practice, useful for moments of anxiety or even to reduce the intensity of a panic attack.

Suggested time: one minute.

INSTRUCTIONS

1. Sit in a comfortable, relaxed position and connect with your breath.

2. With the index, middle, and ring fingers of each hand, softly press the sides of the neck close to the jaw. You should feel the carotid pulse with the fingers of the left hand, and the right hand should be placed at the same height on the right side.

3. Gently massage the neck by circling backward in a calm, continuous motion.

PRECAUTIONS

Contraindications: Low blood pressure.

MEDITATION

Connect with your breathing and heart rate. Feel how the activity of your whole body's functioning slows down. Make the circles slower and slower, and imagine that time itself slows down.

APPLICATIONS

* Stress, anxiety, and trauma
* Neuroendocrine and metabolic regulation

EXERCISE 32: REVERSE BREATHING

This Taoist exercise teaches us that it is beneficial to inhale deeply while simultaneously contracting the abdomen. If done correctly, this exercise adjusts your digestive system and kidneys.

Suggested time: 3 minutes.

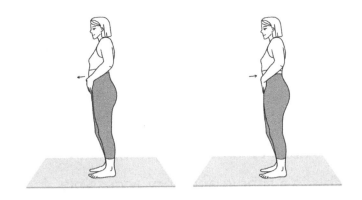

INSTRUCTIONS

1. Stand up with legs at shoulder-width. You can relax your arms, or place both hands open on your belly. Apply a chin lock and focus on the tip of your nose.

2. Inhale deeply and quickly (so that you feel the diaphragm expand) while contracting your abdomen and glutes.

3. Exhale slowly and completely, relaxing the muscles that were contracted on the inhale.

TIPS

Despite inhaling quickly, as you master the practice, you will feel the inhale as a spontaneous pull of the air; it requires no effort and makes no sound. Make sure you perform full diaphragmatic breathing. If not done so, you will be "sending too much fire to the heart" (overstimulating the system) according to qigong's wisdom. Your focus should pay attention to the belly and digestive organs. You may need to practice diaphragmatic breathing before performing this exercise to make sure you breathe fully despite the contraction.

Variation: For a grounding exercise, perform the exercise barefoot, and use the Horseman pose (exercise 17).

PRECAUTIONS

• Practice on an empty stomach.

• Contraindications: pregnancy; menstruation; chronic digestive issues.

• In case of neck injury, consult with your physician before practicing it.

• In case of high blood pressure or heart conditions, consult with your physician, a well-trained qigong teacher, or a traditional Chinese medicine practitioner.

MEDITATION

This breathing is closely related to the principle of yin and yang. It activates and releases energy while also creating a sense of relaxation. Meditate on how paradoxical life can be (for instance, inhaling when you seem to be exhaling due to contraction). You can use this breath to promote dynamism in your life and happily flow. Understand that we are all one. No radicalisms are needed in a happy life.

APPLICATIONS

• Neuroendocrine and metabolic regulation

• Sleep, rest, and vitality

• Mindful focus

EXERCISE 33: KNEELING SPINAL STRETCH

Any contraction of the umbilical point, whether exhaling or not, leads to activation of the vagus nerve and regulation of the parasympathetic system. In addition to stretching the spine and abdomen and improving awareness in the present moment, this exercise uses a powerful variation to stimulate blood oxygenation and metabolic health.

Suggested time: 2 minutes.

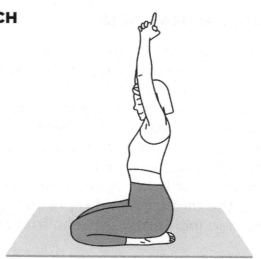

TOOLS

Yoga mat, rolled towel.

INSTRUCTIONS

1. Kneel on your yoga mat. You may need to place a rolled towel under your knees or insteps, respectively. Apply a chin lock. Close your eyes or focus on the tip of your nose.

2. Extend your arms vertically and bring your hands together with interlaced fingers over your head.

3. Inhale fully through the nose and stretch your body up as much as you can.

4. Hold the position for a moment, and then begin contracting your navel in a pumping motion without exhaling for as long as you can.

5. Once you run out of air, exhale fully through the nose.

MEDITATION

Imagine that you sublimate any dense energy you might be holding in the lower spine. Visualize breathing oxygen into every corner of your body as you pump your abdomen.

TIPS

Hold the air out for a few moments before inhaling for a better effect on anxiety.

Variation 1: If the kneeling posture is uncomfortable, sit on the edge of a chair.

Variation 2: Instead of interlacing your fingers, you can also press the palms of your hands together.

Variant 3: Pump your navel in after emptying your lungs. Balance the timing to make the periods of contraction as equal as possible.

PRECAUTIONS

- Practice on an empty stomach.

- Contraindications: Ankle or knee injury; recent abdominal surgery; heart problems; pregnancy; menstruation; chronic digestive conditions.

APPLICATIONS

- Neuroendocrine and metabolic regulation

- Mindful focus

EXERCISE 34: BOW POSE

This is an ideal posture for regulating vagal activity by expanding the abdomen. It can be modified for different levels of flexibility, and it is an essential somatic tool that can help you to release energy and recover vitality, without losing balance. Other benefits of the bow pose are: strengthening the back, opening the chest, adjusting the digestive and reproductive systems, and increasing self-confidence.

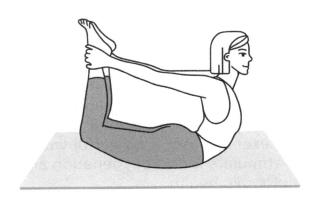

TOOLS

Yoga mat, yoga strap, towel or firm blanket.

INSTRUCTIONS

1. Lie on your stomach with your arms resting at your sides and your legs hip-width apart.

2. As you exhale, bend your knees and bring your heels as close as you can toward your buttocks. Grasp your ankles with your hands.

3. Inhale through the nose while simultaneously lifting your thighs, chest and head. Contract your buttocks to create stability as you lift.

4. Stay in the pose for 30 seconds, if possible. Hold your breath as you feel the stretch in your abdomen.

5. When finished, exhale through the nose as you gently release the posture. Repeat three times.

MEDITATION

Your inner sun expands to fill you with vitality, enthusiasm and self-confidence. Feel your solar plexus both stretching and absorbing energy from the earth. Visualize holding the posture with grace and radiance.

TIPS

Make sure to breathe deeply in the pose by expanding the chest. Hold onto your ankles, not the tops of your feet. Place a firm blanket beneath your hip bones for extra padding, if needed. Do not let your knees splay wider than your hips.

Variation 1: To decrease the challenge, inhale and ascend into the bow pose, and exhale and lower without holding the lift. Inhale and continue with the cycle.

Variation 2: If you can't reach your ankles with your hands, wrap a yoga strap around the front of your ankles before coming into the pose and hold onto the strap as you lift and extend.

PRECAUTIONS

Contraindications: Pregnancy; low back or neck injury; high or low blood pressure; insomnia; migraine.

APPLICATIONS

- Spinal health and flexibility
- Pleasure, joy, and sexual health
- Sleep, rest, and vitality

EXERCISE 35: BOX BREATHING

If you can maintain a sense of balance, you can strengthen and harmonize your body-mind connection. Box breathing, also called 4x4 breathing, can help you maintain balance. The exercise trains the lungs and muscles linked to respiration, adjusts your mood and circadian rhythms, and facilitates a sense of peace and order.

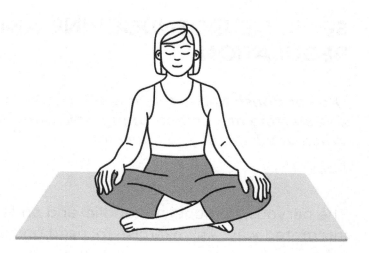

TOOLS

Metronome or breath pacer app.

INSTRUCTIONS

1. Sit in a comfortable position with your chest lifted and expansive. Apply a chin lock. Close your eyes and focus your attention between your eyebrows.

2. Inhale deeply through your nose in a series of four equal inhalations. Hold the air in for four counts. Then exhale through the nose in a series of four equal exhalations.

3. Hold the air out for four counts and repeat the cycle eight to ten times.

TIPS

As you exhale, contract the navel with every stroke. There are breath pacer and metronome apps available to help you count with better precision. To boost the effect on the brain, you can count from 1 to 4 by touching the tips of the index, middle, ring, and little fingers with the tip of the thumb.

PRECAUTIONS

Contraindications: Pregnancy; high blood pressure; lung, heart, or eye problems (choose a relaxed normal breathing instead).

MEDITATION

Everything restores its perfect order and harmony, inside and out.

APPLICATIONS

*   Mindful focus
*   Holistic balance
*   Stress, anxiety, and trauma

SET II. NEUROENDOCRINE AND METABOLIC REGULATION

"Power doesn't have to show off. Power is confident, self-assuring, self-starting and self-stopping, self-warming and self-justifying. When you have it, you know it."

Ralph Ellison

The nervous, immune, metabolic, and endocrine systems function in a very integrated way. Any exercise focused on any one of them will also impact the others. In this exercise, you will work on specific glands that impact digestion and metabolism. Among the glands that will benefit from the exercises in this set are: thyroid, adrenals, pancreas, and liver (although known more as an organ, it has hormone secretion functions, in addition to its direct link to metabolism).

Psycho-emotional causes of imbalance can include communication and assertive listening problems (thyroid); lack of congruence between thoughts, words and actions (thyroid); unresolved feelings of pride (thyroid), fear or guilt (adrenals), and anger or helplessness (liver). You might also be experiencing low self-esteem, need for approval, or feelings of submissiveness (pancreas).

Somatic exercises that focus on metabolic regulation and neuroendocrine function can improve digestion, relieve heartburn and stomach imbalances, reduce stress reactivity, restore vitality, and ultimately improve mood and self-confidence.

TIPS FOR A HEALTHY LIFESTYLE

- Hydrate with room temperature water.
- Practice intermittent fasting (consultation with a specialist is suggested).
- Exercise regularly.
- Eat slowly.

NEUROENDOCRINE AND METABOLIC REGULATION

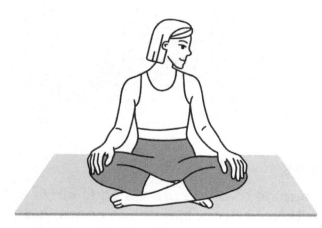

NECK ROLLS

THREE TO FIVE TIMES IN
EACH DIRECTION

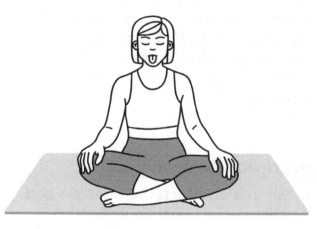

PANTING DOG BREATH

1 - 3 MINUTES

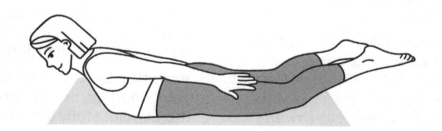

LOCUST POSE

REPEAT THREE TIMES

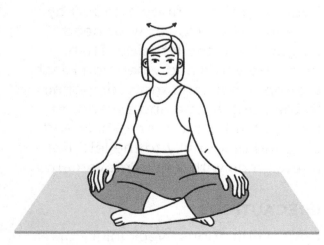

TORSO TWIST

REPEAT FIVE TO TEN TIMES

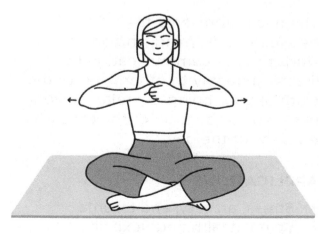

BEAR GRIP

REPEAT AS MANY TIMES AS NEEDED

EXERCISE 36: NECK ROLLS

This is a common and effective exercise for alleviating neck tension. This area contains the thyroid, a gland that regulates metabolism and other essential functions. With this exercise you also oxygenate the brain and adjust the functioning of the pituitary gland.

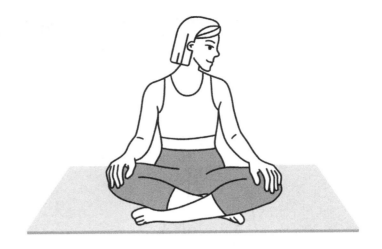

INSTRUCTIONS

1. Sit in a comfortable position and allow your chest to expand.

2. Bring your chin toward your neck, and inhale as you slowly roll your head to the left. Bring your left ear toward the left shoulder then roll back to center.

3. Exhale as your head rolls to the right, and your right ear comes toward your right shoulder. Repeat slowly, rolling your chin toward your chest and your ear toward your shoulder, three to five times in each direction.

MEDITATION

The neck represents the bridge between body, mind, and spirit. Nurture your communication by listening deeply to others and to the truth of your being. By relaxing your neck, you also let go of the excessive burdens of the day.

APPLICATIONS

- Stress, anxiety, and trauma
- Spinal health and flexibility

TIPS

Imagine that you draw a wide circle with your nose. Maintain a controlled movement and do not let the head collapse as it goes back.

Variation 1: "Say no" by moving your head to the left on the inhale and to the right on the exhale. Maintain a continuous motion that is attentive to stretching with gentleness.

Variation 2: "Say yes" by moving your head up on the inhale and down the exhale. Maintain a continuous motion that is attentive to stretching with gentleness.

Variation 3: Move your head in a figure eight (or infinity symbol) by exhaling as you lower your head diagonally to the left side. Then, inhale upwards and when you reach the top exhale and move diagonally to the right. Inhale and ascend on the right side, and then exhale and descend diagonally to the left. Repeat a few times with a fluid movement.

PRECAUTIONS

Contraindications: Neck injury or compression; high or low blood pressure; dizziness and migraine; severe osteoporosis; brain tumors.

EXERCISE 37: PANTING DOG BREATH

The breathing exercise is a simple and effective therapeutic tool. Panting dog breath consists of sticking out your tongue while breathing. It benefits the body's metabolism and thermoregulation, releases toxins, and relaxes the vocal cords.

Suggested time: 1 to 3 minutes.

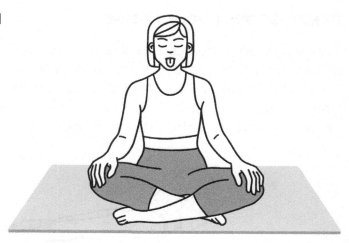

INSTRUCTIONS

1. Sit in a comfortable upright position, with your chest lifted and open. Apply a chin lock and close your eyes while directing your gaze inwardly toward the forehead.

2. Open your mouth wide and stick your tongue out.

3. Pant through the mouth at a dynamic pace, about two breaths per second. Contract the navel briefly on every exhale.

4. Do it for as long as you need, and then close your mouth. Inhale fully through the nose. Hold in for a couple of seconds, and exhale fully.

TIPS

The more you stick the tongue out, the better the effect on the thyroid and metabolism. It's okay if you cough during the exercise. Drinking water is recommended after finishing the exercise to assist in the elimination of toxins.

Variation 1: To boost the detox effect, perform the "breath of fire" by closing your mouth and breathing through the nose with the same pattern.

Variation 2: To decrease the challenge, breathe through the mouth with the tongue out, but keep a normal breathing pattern. If pregnant, do not contract your navel.

MEDITATION

Imagine that you burn all the toxins in your body and expel them through your mouth. Visualize that with each breath you heal your liver and release accumulated anger.

PRECAUTIONS

- Practice with an empty stomach.

- Contraindications: Digestive problems; cirrhosis or severe liver problems.

APPLICATIONS

- Stress, anxiety, and trauma
- Mindful focus

EXERCISE 38: LOCUST POSE

This yoga posture adjusts the kidneys and adrenal glands, which are in charge of producing the stress hormones adrenaline, noradrenaline and cortisol. Thus, this balance directly helps in regulating stress response and recovering balance in mind and body. It also stimulates the digestive and reproductive systems, and stretches the core body and legs.

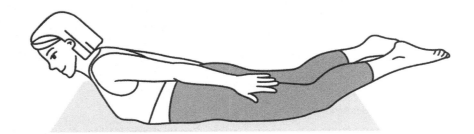

TOOLS

Yoga mat or comfortable surface, bolster, blanket.

INSTRUCTIONS

1. Lie down on your stomach with arms relaxed at a 45-degree angle away from the sides. Rotate your hands so your palms face down.

2. Pull your legs up by squeezing the buttocks, pelvic floor, and thighs.

3. Inhale as you lift the chest, neck, head, and arms off of the floor. Keep shoulders relaxed as part of the chest opening.

4. Hold the pose and take a few breaths through the nose before returning slowly to the starting position.

5. Rest for a few moments then repeat three times.

TIPS

You may need to place a rolled blanket or a bolster under your thighs. A rolled blanket under your ribcage or hips may also be helpful.

PRECAUTIONS

Contraindications: Pregnancy and menstruation; kidney problems; high blood pressure; recent abdominal surgery; low back problems or injury.

MEDITATION

The kidneys accumulate guilt and fear of being yourself and taking real initiative in your life. Recognize, accept, and expel any similar feelings from you with this exercise.

APPLICATIONS

- Sleep, health, and vitality
- Stress, anxiety, and trauma
- Spinal health and flexibility

EXERCISE 39: TORSO TWIST

Stomach health, while highly dependent on what you ingest, can also be addressed through conscious breathing and movement. This exercise can help to alleviate heartburn and reflux, massage inner organs, and promote spinal health.

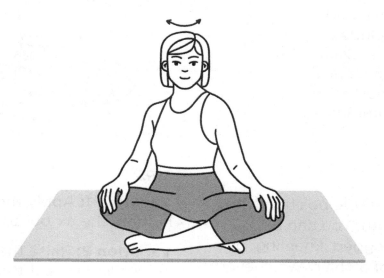

INSTRUCTIONS

1. Sit in a comfortable position with legs crossed, or on the edge of a chair. Apply a chin lock, open the chest and place your hands on your knees.

2. Inhale through the nose and hold the inhalation while squeezing the pelvic floor and twisting the torso in one direction while keeping the head looking directly forward; twist in the opposite direction and then exhale back to center.

3. Repeat five to ten times.

TIPS

Manage your air holding capacity in order to twist in both directions on a single breath.

PRECAUTIONS

- Practice on an empty stomach.

- Contraindications: Heart problems; neck or spine injury; pregnancy; dizziness or migraine; severe stomach problems.

MEDITATION

Feel everything inside your body that you have been ignoring. Imagine oxygen reaching the stomach, regulating the pH, and healing heartburn.

APPLICATIONS

- Spinal health and flexibility
- Stress, anxiety, and trauma
- Vagus nerve regulation

EXERCISE 40: BEAR GRIP

This pose is a great middle back pain reliever and also works to relieve any tension that has accumulated in your arms, chest, and shoulders. We include it here as it has a stimulant effect on the thymus gland, which is very important to keep a powerful immune system.

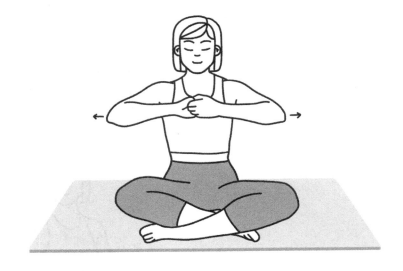

INSTRUCTIONS

1. Sit in a comfortable position with your chest open. You can be sitting cross-legged, kneeling, or on the edge of a chair—whichever feels most comfortable. Apply a chin lock and close your eyes.

2. Bring both arms in front of your chest, parallel to the ground.

3. Open both palms in front of each other. The right palm faces you and the left one faces outwards. The hands grasp each other, as if forming a yin and yang.

4. Inhale through the nose and hold the inhalation; try to pull the hands apart while you squeeze the pelvic floor. Use maximum force for as long as you can hold your breath; feel the tension in your arms and back. Keep arms parallel to the ground at heart height.

5. Exhale through the mouth as you relax the tension, but do not undo the grip. Repeat as many times as needed.

TIPS

Variation 1: Apply the grip while holding the air out too.

Variation 2: Raise the grip at neck height and repeat the exercise. The effect will focus on the neck and thyroid gland.

PRECAUTIONS

Contraindications: High blood pressure; wrist or shoulder injury.

MEDITATION

Imagine your strength boosting your immune system. The tensions accumulated in your arms and chest related to resentment, stress, and self-limiting thoughts can vanish.

APPLICATIONS

- Stress, anxiety, and trauma
- Spinal health and flexibility

SET III. PLEASURE, JOY, AND SEXUAL HEALTH

"It's time we saw sex as the truly sacred art that it is. A deep meditation, a holy communion and a dance with the force of creation."

Marcus Allen

What is the point of living a healthy, conscious life if we are not happy? Enjoying life is an essential part of health, and that is why this specific set focuses on experiencing a full array of physical and emotional pleasures.

The experience of joy connects to dopamine and serotonin secretion, microbiome and intestinal health, the reproductive system (including the secretion of stress regulating hormones like oxytocin and estrogen), and the lower back and hips (which can be connected to imbalances in the adrenal and reproductive organs).

Psycho-emotional causes of imbalance can include depression, trauma, sexual abuse, miscarriages, grief, shame, guilt, and unresolved feelings or trauma related to identity, gender, and sexual orientation.

Somatic exercises that focus on supporting a sense of well-being and pleasure can improve self-esteem, vitality, creativity, and initiative. It can also relieve lower back pain, hip pain, and sinus congestion.

TIPS FOR A HEALTHY LIFESTYLE

- Exercise regularly.

- Eat a variety of whole foods including fruit, vegetables, fermented foods and vinaigrettes to improve your intestinal microbiome.

- Avoid dairy products.

- Walk in the sun and practice hobbies and pleasurable activities.

- Reduce exposure to screens and artificial lights, especially when waking up and at night.

- Build healthy interpersonal boundaries, and only engage in consensual sexual activity that feels good for your sense of well-being.

PLEASURE, JOY, AND SEXUAL HEALTH

HIP TWIST

REPEAT TEN TIMES IN EACH DIRECTION

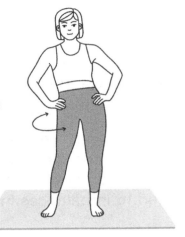

QIGONG EXERCISE FOR GONADIC HEALTH

1 MINUTE PER SIDE

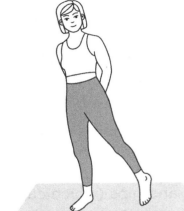

HUMMING BEE BREATH

REPEAT FIVE TO TEN TIMES

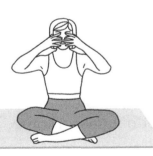

"LA..." MEDITATION

REPEAT AS MANY TIMES AS NEEDED

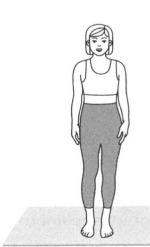

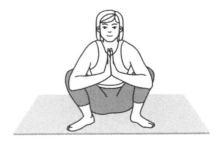

FROG POSE

1 - 2 MINUTES

EXERCISE 41: HIP TWIST

This is an easy exercise for stretching and relaxing the hips. When performed consciously, hip twists massage your digestive and reproductive organs, tone muscles, and enhance sexual pleasure.

INSTRUCTIONS

1. Stand upright, with your legs a little wider than shoulder width apart. Place your hands on your waist. Apply a chin lock and perform slow, wide circles with your hips while keeping your head still.

2. Inhale through your nose as you rotate forward, and exhale through your mouth as you rotate backward.

3. Repeat ten times in each direction.

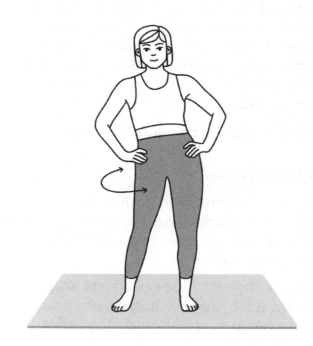

TIPS

Inhale and exhale as fully as possible.

Variation 1: Perform the twists while holding the air in.

PRECAUTIONS

Contraindications: After hip replacement; back or hip injury. Variation 1 is contraindicated for pregnancy or heart problems.

MEDITATION

Remember that you deserve to enjoy life, you deserve to be creative and express the real self.

APPLICATIONS

• Spinal health and flexibility

• Grounding and sciatic nerve health

EXERCISE 42: QIGONG EXERCISE FOR GONADIC HEALTH

The health of our gonads and reproductive system is important for sexual health and enjoyment, as well as for assertive stress management. This qigong exercise is a direct message to both the ovaries and prostate and functions as a general tension reliever. It also benefits the lumbar region of the back and pelvic floor.

Suggested time: 1 minute per side.

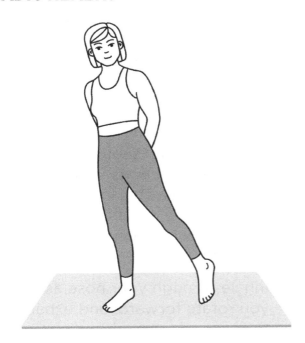

INSTRUCTIONS

1. Stand upright with your feet shoulder-width apart. Grasp your hands behind your low back in a relaxed way.

2. Move the left foot outwards and form a 90-degree angle with your feet. Your torso should also point to the left.

3. Inhale, and then exhale through the nose as you squeeze your right buttock and stretch your right foot at the same time. This will tilt your body forward, loading your left leg with most of the weight. Feel how your whole right leg stretches with the movement.

4. Inhale through your nose as you now stretch the left leg and foot while relaxing the right leg (this will tilt your body in the opposite direction).

5. Continue for one minute. It's a fluid movement: tilt back and forth like a metronome.

6. Return to the center, and change sides. Bring the left foot parallel to the right foot, rotate the left foot outward 90-degree angle, and then tilt the torso in the same direction.

TIPS

Concentrate on fully stretching the leg in each movement. As you contract your glute on the exhale, feel the firm pressure coming from below into your pelvic floor and internal organs.

PRECAUTIONS

Contraindications: Ovarian or prostate health problems; low back or hip injury; pregnancy.

MEDITATION

Both sex and happiness in life depend on knowing how to flow. This easy back-and-forth exercise is an excellent reminder of your ability to flow.

APPLICATIONS

- Stress, anxiety, and trauma

- Neuroendocrine and metabolic regulation

EXERCISE 43: HUMMING BEE BREATH

This breathing exercise relieves stress and evokes joy. By blocking all your senses, it invites you to go inwards. The resonance produced by breathing generates a neural and endocrine adjustment, relaxes the face, and relieves headaches and sinusitis.

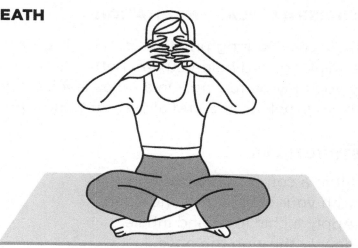

INSTRUCTIONS

1. Sit in a comfortable position with your chest lifted and open. Apply a chin lock, close your eyes, and focus your gaze inward toward the forehead.

2. Block your ears with your thumbs. Rest your index fingers on your closed eyes. Your middle fingers should lightly block the nostrils while your ring and little fingers rest above and below the closed mouth, respectively.

3. Inhale fully through the nose (you may need to release the pressure from the middle fingers for this) and make a sonorous "M" sound.

4. Once you run out of air, hold for a few seconds and then repeat five to ten times while allowing yourself to relax.

APPLICATIONS

• Mindful focus
• Spinal health and flexibility
• Sleep, rest, and vitality

TIPS

If you keep the chin lock properly, you will feel the resonance through the whole spine. That will boost its effect on the nervous system. The partial block of the nostrils is important to "enclose" the sound within your head.

Variation 1: Block your ears with the thumbs only.

PRECAUTIONS

• Practice on an empty stomach.

• In case of heart diseases, practice it with no breath retention.

• Do not practice while laying down.

• Contraindications: Active ear infection; low or very high blood pressure

MEDITATION

Let this breathwork inspire you to resonate with others through the joy and radiant expression of your soul. You deserve to share the light of your heart and be happy.

EXERCISE 44: "LA..." MEDITATION

This simple chanting practice can cut through both resentments and overthinking, and help you feel better. It also leads you to release any self-pity you may be feeling. On a reflex level, the relaxation in the jaw will also relax your pelvic area and allow you to flow better with your emotions.

INSTRUCTIONS

1. Sit in a comfortable position with your chest lifted and open. Apply a chin lock, and inhale deeply through the nose.

2. Chant "La...". Open your mouth wide without forcing it. Try to make the sound last for as long as possible while also staying relaxed.

3. Repeat as many times as needed. Once finished, keep meditating in silence.

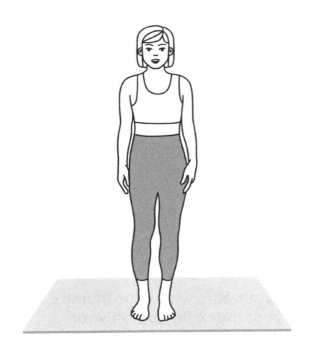

TIPS

You may notice how your mouth opens more and more after each repetition. You may want to keep the mouth wide open or yawn.

MEDITATION

Open your heart to happiness, bliss, and peace. This practice may seem ridiculous, but it is effective. Overcome self-pity and enjoy it.

APPLICATIONS

• Stress, anxiety, and trauma
• Sleep, rest, and vitality

EXERCISE 45: FROG POSE

Sedentary lifestyles have distanced most of us from some postural habits that were once common, like sitting in frog posture, which around the world is used in many situations like cooking in front of a campfire, or even during labor. This is an excellent posture that opens the hips, and elongates the spine; it is ideal for pregnant women with precautions. It helps to counteract the effects of a sedentary lifestyle and even prevent its impact, as you can practice it before sitting down to work.

Suggested time: 1 to 2 minutes.

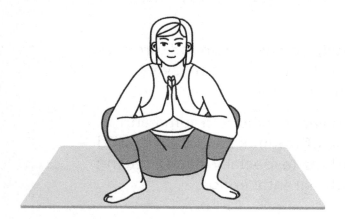

TIPS

Keep the position of your elbows actively pressing against your inner thighs in order to help your back remain straight and deepen the stretch.

Variation 1: Place a yoga block or low chair under your buttocks for stability.

TOOLS

Yoga mat, and yoga block or low chair for easier variations.

PRECAUTIONS

Contraindications: Low back or knee pain; hip injury or recent surgery.

INSTRUCTIONS

1. Stand upright, with your feet slightly wider than shoulder-width apart, pointing out at a 45-degree angle.

2. Inhale, and as you exhale, bend your knees and sit into the pose, with your hands in prayer position and your forearms parallel to the floor to help you maintain the balance and openness of the pose.

3. Stay in the posture and breathe deeply. To finish, rise on an inhale.

MEDITATION

Open your hips. Connect with your instincts. Absorb the force of the earth directly through your pelvic floor. If your posture makes you tired or tingly, focus on taking care of your alignment and sending oxygen to that area.

APPLICATIONS

* Grounding and sciatic nerve health
* Spinal health and flexibility

SET IV. HOLISTIC BALANCE

"Happiness is not a matter of intensity but of balance and order and rhythm and harmony."

Thomas Merton

Stress and balance can be opposing forces. Therefore, cultivating a deep balance in life will allow you to be more resilient in the face of life's challenges. Part of that balance can be supported in the neuroendocrine system and brain activity, and deepened by working on body awareness and balance.

Somatic exercises that cultivate balance help to calm the mind, promote mood regulation and develop discernment. They can also relieve headaches, and help with back health and flexibility.

The main psycho-emotional causes of imbalance include trauma and lack of embodiment (dissociation) because of trauma; lack of order and prioritization; imbalances in circadian rhythms (especially sleep); feeling lost or disoriented in life; and conflicts with parental image.

TIPS FOR A HEALTHY LIFESTYLE

- Take time to regularly enjoy nature and absorb sunlight.

- Practice physical exercise that focuses on body awareness, and cognitive exercise that focuses on mindful attention and neuroplasticity.

- Consume foods that promote brain health: Omega-3 fatty acids (EPA and DHA), zinc, vitamin D, and magnesium.

HOLISTIC BALANCE

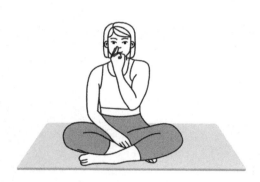

ALTERNATE NOSTRIL BREATHING

2 - 3 MINUTES

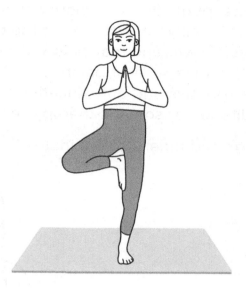

YOGA TREE POSE

1 - 2 MINUTES
PER SIDE

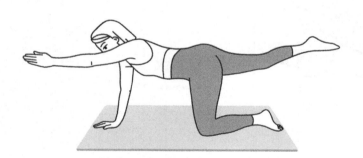

**ALTERNATE LEG
AND ARM STRETCHES**

1 - 3 MINUTES

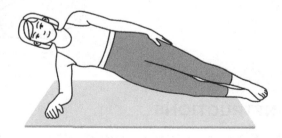

SIDE PLANK

HOLD THE SIDE PLANK POSITION AND
BREATHE FOR A FEW BREATHS, THEN
EXHALE AND RELEASE TO THE GROUND

REPEAT ON BOTH SIDES

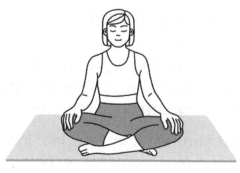

**OCULAR EXERCISE FOR
BRAIN ADJUSTMENT**

3 MINUTES

EXERCISE 46: ALTERNATE NOSTRIL BREATHING

This is a classic yoga breathing technique called Nadi Shodhana, which means "purification of energy channels." It can create a profound balancing effect on all your systems. At the psycho-emotional level, it is a powerful stress reliever and may help you compassionately overcome trauma. At the physiological level, it balances the brain and nervous system, and boosts anti-oxidative and detoxification functions. It is a great practice before any meditation or somatic therapy session.

Suggested time: 2 to 3 minutes.

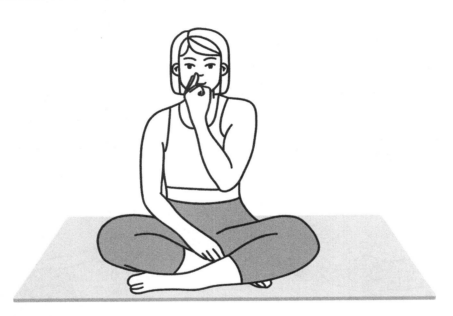

INSTRUCTIONS

1. Sit in a comfortable position with your chest lifted and open. Your eyes can be closed, or focused on your forehead.

2. Rest one hand on your lap and use the other hand to press one nostril closed; then inhale through the open nostril.

3. Release the blocked nostril as you alternate and close the other nostril, and exhale and then inhale.

4. Release the blocked nostril as you alternate and close the other side again, exhale, and then inhale, and continue in this alternating pattern of blocking one side and then breathing in and out.

5. To finish, release your hand and rest it in your lap. Inhale deeply through both nostrils and hold. After a few moments, exhale and relax.

TIPS

The pressure of the fingertips on the blocked nostril should seal the nostril completely, but still feel relaxed. Try to use the thumb and the little finger for the blocks so that it is easy to rotate your hand and alternate which nostril you are blocking. For instance, the thumb of the right hand blocks the right nostril and the right little finger rotates to block the left nostril. *Change the block before the exhale.*

Variation 1: Hold the air in or out as you prefer (not suggested in case of heart problems), but take the same time for each part of the breathing cycle.

Variation 2: Slow down the breathing cycle for a deeper effect.

PRECAUTIONS

Practice on an empty stomach.

MEDITATION

See yourself in balance with mind, body, and emotions. Your life becomes a constant, harmonic flow. This breathing seems easy, but it demands attention to keep doing the nostril shift correctly. That same thing happens with life and the thoughts we give force to: we need to stay aware of ourselves and our breathing to maintain balance.

APPLICATIONS

- Mindful focus
- Neuroendocrine and metabolic regulation
- Stress, anxiety, and trauma

EXERCISE 47: YOGA TREE POSE

This is a classical pose for balance. Despite being taught to beginners, it is a bit harder than it looks, but with discipline and thoughtfulness you can find your balance. This is a great exercise to cultivate holistic balance and body awareness, while having some fun learning it. It strengthens the core and legs, opens the hips, stretches inner thigh and groin muscles, and grounds your energy.

Suggested time: 1 to 2 minutes per side.

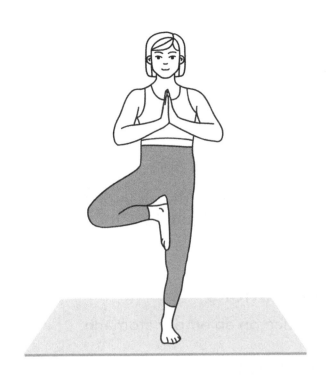

INSTRUCTIONS

1. Stand up tall with heels together. Roll your shoulders back and down to open your chest. Apply a chin lock and bring your hands together in prayer pose with your forearms parallel to the ground.

2. Gaze at the floor in front of you to help keep your balance.

3. Raise your right foot and rest the sole of the right foot on the left thigh or calf (not on the knee). The right knee points to the side.

4. Engage your core, breathe deeply, and focus on keeping your balance.

5. When finished, release the right foot, rest briefly, and repeat on the other side.

APPLICATIONS

- Grounding and sciatic nerve health
- Pleasure, joy, and sexual health

TIPS

You can use your hand to place your foot against your thigh. Avoid resting the foot on the knee, so that you don't put pressure on the joint. Make sure that your raised knee energetically points outwards; it will help you find your center and stay balanced. You can practice close to a wall if you would like to place your hand against it for support.

Variation: To ease stability, extend your arms out to the side parallel to the floor. Keep fingers straight and together.

PRECAUTIONS

Contraindications: Ankle, knee, or hip injury.

MEDITATION

The balance in life is grounded in your roots in the earth. Your firmness and ability to focus are what really matters. Visualize yourself as strong, healthy, and as flexible as a tree.

EXERCISE 48: ALTERNATE LEG AND ARM STRETCHES

This exercise promotes bilateral brain integration, spinal alignment, and balance. It strengthens the core and back of the shoulders, and helps with kidney, reproductive, and heart health.

Suggested time: 1 to 3 minutes.

TOOLS

Yoga mat, knee pad or blankets.

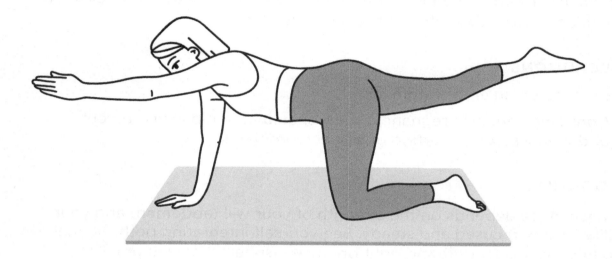

INSTRUCTIONS

1. Kneel on all fours with your hands and knees aligned under your shoulders and hips, respectively. Apply a chin lock and keep the head and spine neutral. Spread your fingers for more balance.

2. Engage the core (abdomen, buttocks, and pelvic floor) as you inhale and extend your left arm and right leg. Point your fingers to the front. Contract your buttocks and raise the extended leg to torso level or slightly above.

3. Exhale as you return to the starting position, then inhale and repeat with the opposite arm and leg.

TIPS

Practice barefoot to avoid the extra weight of shoes. Fingers spread at the starting position gives you more balance, but if you press the fingers together when you extend it will promote brain synchronization and focus.

Variation 1: For extra cushion, place a blanket under your hands and knees.

Variation 2: To increase the challenge, instead of returning to starting position on an exhale pull your arm and leg close to the core, curve your spine, and tuck your head. Repeat the movement: extend your arm and leg out, hold, and then pull your arm and leg in close to the core for a few repetitions before switching to the other side.

PRECAUTIONS

- Practice on an empty stomach.
- Contraindications: Pregnancy; knee, shoulder, or hip injury; recent abdominal surgery; vertigo or balance problems.

MEDITATION

Balance in life depends on the strength of your will (abdomen) and your ability to stay focused and steady. See yourself integrating both rational and intuitive minds (left and right brain hemispheres) as you practice steady strength.

APPLICATIONS

- Spinal health and flexibility
- Mindful alert and focus
- Neuroendocrine and metabolic regulation

EXERCISE 49: SIDE PLANK

This exercise focuses on the oblique abdominals and in their work in the abdominal area to adjust the colon and strengthen hips, arms, and back.

TOOLS

Yoga mat, yoga block, bolster.

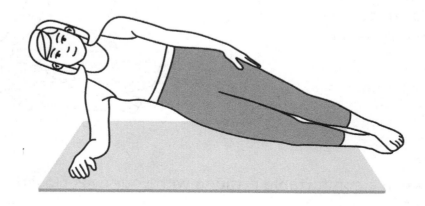

INSTRUCTIONS

1. Lie on your right side with your legs extended. Use your right forearm to support the weight of your torso. Place your right hand on the ground and point it to the front. Rest your left arm along the left side of your body.

2. Inhale, and then as you exhale lift your hips off the ground to create a straight diagonal line from your feet to your head. (Your right hand, forearm, and right foot are the only parts of your body in contact with the ground.)

3. Hold the side plank position and breathe for a few breaths, then exhale and release to the ground. Repeat on both sides.

APPLICATIONS

- Spinal health and flexibility
- Mindful alert and focus
- Sleep, rest, and vitality

TIPS

Engage your core and activate the muscles in your legs to maintain the pose and stabilize your lower back.

Variation 1: Place a blanket or yoga block under your leg for support.

Variation 2: Straighten the arm on which you are supporting the weight and hold the posture. You can also stretch the opposite arm vertically.

PRECAUTIONS

Contraindications: Recent abdominal surgery; pregnancy; strain in your neck, shoulders, or any other joints; neck, arm, shoulder, or ankle injury. Consult your doctor in case of prosthesis.

MEDITATION

Feel how your willpower is strengthened and refined. Let this exercise enhance your character, grounding, and self-control.

EXERCISE 50: OCULAR EXERCISE FOR BRAIN ADJUSTMENT

The following exercise is a little trick that adjusts your brain and endocrine activity. It can mitigate headaches, including migraines. It also works to lower blood pressure, relieve stress, gain focus, and even help you fall asleep.

Suggested time: 3 minutes.

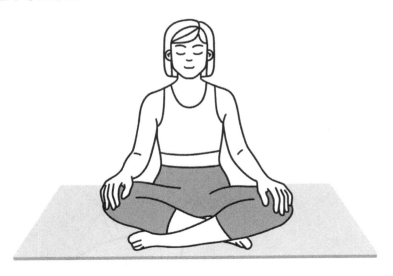

INSTRUCTIONS

1. Sit or lie down in a comfortable position with your eyes closed.

2. Focus your gaze in and up, as if you are looking toward the crown of your head from the inside.

3. Breathe deeply and do nothing else. You will feel a pressure above your eyeballs but it is normal and may fade over time.

TIPS

If you are experiencing a headache or migraine, continue the exercise for at least 5 minutes. Turn lights off and avoid screens for a while after finishing the exercise. Let your eyes and brain rest.

Variation: Put gentle pressure on your eyelids with the palms of your hands.

PRECAUTIONS

Contraindications: Low blood pressure; glaucoma.

MEDITATION

Imagine that you are pressing a "reset" button in your brain and your consciousness: it will slow thoughts down and remind you not to ruminate.

APPLICATIONS

- Neuroendocrine and metabolic regulation

- Sleep, rest, and vitality

- Stress, anxiety, and trauma

SET V. MINDFUL FOCUS

"Just remember that those things that get attention flourish."

Victoria Moran

Attention and concentration problems are becoming more and more frequent, due to the distractions of modern technology and new sources of stress. And it is also true that, in such changing times, some people experience the emergence of intuitive talents that need to be integrated. Studies show that lack of motivation or emotional connection can contribute to concentration and memory problems. Somatic exercises can help you to take care of these aspects in your life, and strengthen your capacity to feel focused, alert, and resilient.

Common causes of psycho-emotional imbalance include depression, anxiety, difficulty with self-regulation, imbalances in circadian rhythms (especially sleep), and a feeling of disconnection from life purpose and sense of priorities.

The benefits of mindful focus include: improved mood regulation, rest and healing for the eyes, increased self-confidence and motivation, and a more grounded intuition and assertive decision-making.

TIPS FOR A HEALTHY LIFESTYLE

- Practice activities that you enjoy.

- Express your emotions.

- Attend psychotherapy to heal trauma, and become more self-aware.

- Consume foods that promote brain and neurological health: Omega-3 fatty acids (EPA and DHA), zinc, vitamin D, magnesium.

- Reduce your exposure to screens, especially in the early morning and evening hours.

- Avoid foods that contribute to inflammation (including gluten, dairy, and refined sugar) or irritate the nervous system, (including monosodium glutamate, aspartame, salt, and artificial flavoring).

MINDFUL FOCUS

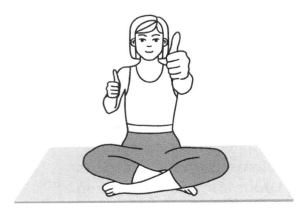

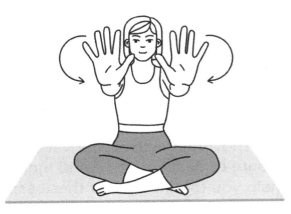

EXERCISE FOR EYE HEALTH
2 - 3 MINUTES

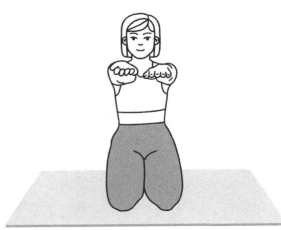

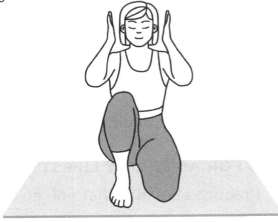

NEUTRAL MIND AND DISCERNMENT
3 - 5 MINUTES

TO DEVELOP A GROUNDED INTUITION
2 - 5 MINUTES

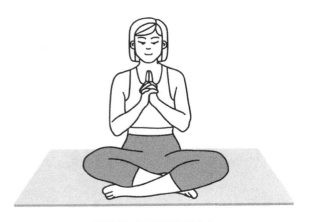

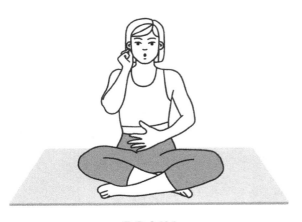

THE ANTENNA
3 - 5 MINUTES

BRAIN SYNCHRONIZATION
2 - 3 MINUTES

EXERCISE 51: EXERCISE FOR EYE HEALTH

This series for eye health counteracts some of the strain from digital screens, activates the oculocardiac reflex, alleviates the effects of eye fatigue, and triggers a parasympathetic reaction that promotes relaxation.

Suggested time: one minute per movement.

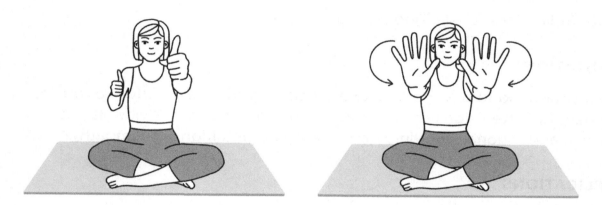

INSTRUCTIONS

1. Bring your arms straight out in front at shoulder height, parallel to each other. Apply a chin lock and focus your eyes forward and to the center.

2. Raise your thumbs up in front of your eyes and gaze toward the center, with your peripheral gaze on your nails. Stretch the thumb of one hand straight out in front and bring the other one close to your face. Keep your peripheral gaze on both nails and you start to alternately move your hands back and forth (from stretched out in front, then close to your face). Rest with your eyes closed.

3. Open your hands with your palms facing to the front. Inhale as you move arms outwards and exhale as you bring them to the center (keep them straight). Keep your peripheral gaze on both hands. Rest with your eyes closed.

4. Hands open with palms facing to the front. Keep your peripheral gaze on both hands while making wide circles with your hands. Rest with your eyes closed.

5. Select one point close to you and another one further away. Alternate your focus between both targets, but do not move your head. Perform the exercise for 30 to 60 seconds, and then relax with your eyes closed.

TIPS

Avoid blinking. Eyes remain focused forward and to the center in all exercises (excepting for the last step). Rest your eyes after the exercise and avoid exposure to screens and intense lights for a few minutes.

PRECAUTIONS

Contraindications: Low blood pressure; glaucoma.

MEDITATION

Open your mind to new perspectives, including the perspectives of others. Eye damage often signifies resistance to flexing one's worldview. Is your physical and rational sight in balance with your intuition and empathy?

APPLICATIONS

• Stress, anxiety, and trauma
• Self-love and emotional awareness

EXERCISE 52: NEUTRAL MIND AND DISCERNMENT

Neutral mind refers to the ability to perceive both the internal (emotions, thoughts) and external stimuli without prejudice. It is mainly associated with the frontal lobe, and developing this skill allows us to make decisions with true freedom. However, this is one of the functions that can become inhibited with chronic stress and trauma. When this happens, we stop making decisions (even if we think we do) and we only react or respond in a conditioned way. This exercise awakens mental alertness and stimulates the frontal lobe. In this way you can reduce prejudices and make more discerning choices.

Suggested time: 3 to 5 minutes.

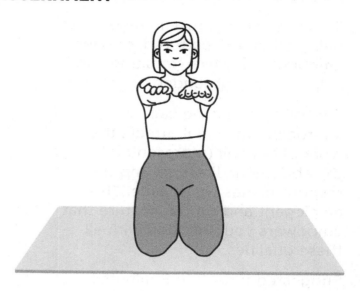

TOOLS

Yoga mat or chair, blanket, knee pad, or cushion.

INSTRUCTIONS

1. Sit in a kneeling pose on the yoga mat (or sit on the edge of a chair). Keep your spine straight and your chest open.

2. Apply a chin lock and raise both arms forward at shoulder height.

3. Press your hands firmly together with the right palm facing up and your left palm facing down.

4. Breathe deeply in the posture. Keep eyes open and staring at a fixed point. Avoid blinking.

5. To finish, inhale deeply and hold the posture for a few moments. Exhale and relax with eyes closed.

TIPS

The longer the better. If you keep the correct arm alignment, you can adjust your nervous system. You may grow tired after a couple of minutes, but it's a very healing resource for your mind to practice for five to ten minutes.

Variation 1: To boost detoxification and mental alertness, use the panting dog breath during the exercise.

PRECAUTIONS

Contraindications: Variation 1 should not be performed when pregnant, or if you have digestive problems, cirrhosis, or liver problems.

MEDITATION

Imagine that you're opening both your physical and intuitive eyes. This practice, especially if including the panting dog breath, develops full awareness in the here and now.

APPLICATIONS

- Holistic balance
- Sleep, rest, and vitality

EXERCISE 53: TO DEVELOP A GROUNDED INTUITION

Some people confuse intuition with being ethereal, scattered, or overly emotional. However, intuition can help you stay grounded.

Part of it is what we call interoception, and it affects the work of our will (represented by the abdomen), lifestyle, and the responsibilities we assume. This is an elegant and simple posture that empowers your intuition with all these qualities.

Suggested time: 2 to 5 minutes.

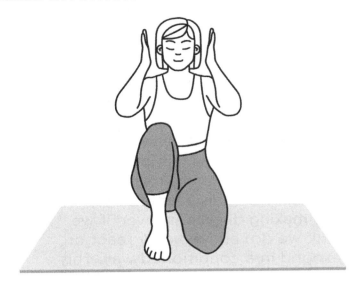

TOOLS

Yoga mat, blanket, chair.

INSTRUCTIONS

1. Sit in a kneeling position on your left heel. Rest your right foot on the floor so that the knee is bent in front of your chest. Keep your torso vertical and chest open.

2. Place your hands open at the sides of your head, so that palms are aligned with your ears. Eyes focused on the tip of the nose.

3. Begin breathing deeply. Imagine that you have a halo of energy around your head that is becoming harmonized as you breathe.

APPLICATIONS

- Grounding and sciatic nerve health
- Self-love and emotional awareness

TIPS

Use a knee pad or blanket under your buttocks, or between the instep and the floor. If the posture is uncomfortable, you can take a kneeling position with both heels tucked beneath you, or sit on the edge of a chair.

PRECAUTIONS

- Contraindications: Ankle or knee injury.

- If pregnant, consult with your physician before performing the kneeling posture.

MEDITATION

Imagine yourself as an antenna that is grounded; feel your electromagnetic field finding balance and sharpening your intuition.

EXERCISE 54: THE ANTENNA

This exercise builds on the previous one, and expands that grounding to let you connect with your heart and surroundings.

This antenna meditation is a nice resource to develop empathy with yourself and others. The eye focus helps to develop emotional awareness.

Suggested time: 3 to 5 minutes.

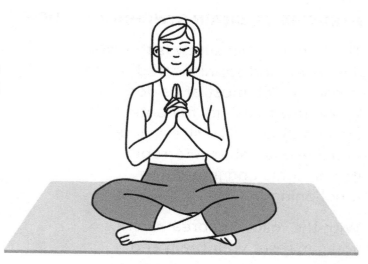

TOOLS

Zafu, cushion, or chair.

INSTRUCTIONS

1. Sit in a comfortable position with your chest open. Apply a chin lock and bring your hands together in front of your chest; interlace your fingers and relax your elbows.

2. Extend your index fingers so they point up together, and your fingertips are just below throat level.

3. Focus your gaze on the tips of the index fingers and breathe deeply. Imagine your fingers as an antenna with which you can scan your heart and all of your surroundings.

TIPS

Ideally, sit crossed-legged on the ground, to open the pelvic area and create a feeling of groundedness. If you feel strain in your back, or if your knees are above your hip level, sit on a cushion or in a chair. Use this meditation as a resource for scanning your body. Pay attention to any pain or discomfort in your body and deepen your awareness to gain insight into the emotional and spiritual background of the pain.

MEDITATION

Perceive everything as an extension and projection of yourself.

APPLICATIONS

• Self-love and emotional awareness
• Stress and anxiety
• Sleep, rest, and vitality

EXERCISE 55: BRAIN SYNCHRONIZATION

The human brain surely is the most advanced and sophisticated organ in nature. Yet, most of us don't know how to use its full potential. Many problems like stress and bad lifestyle habits interrupt its harmonic and integrated functioning.

With the following breathwork, you can reset your brain and stimulate it to work in harmony. Additionally, Eastern traditions suggest that a pressure point in your ear can stimulate brain function.

Suggested time: 2 to 3 minutes.

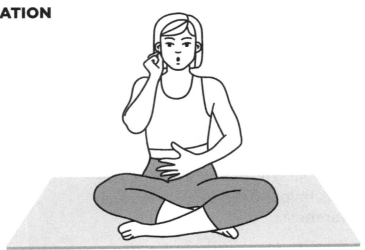

INSTRUCTIONS

1. Sit comfortably with your chest lifted and open. Apply a chin lock, place your left hand on your belly, and close your eyes.

2. With the index and thumb fingers of your right hand, firmly press both sides of your right earlobe.

3. Open your mouth just a little (like if you were going to sip from a straw).

4. Inhale and exhale through the mouth, ideally producing a whistling sound both on the inhale and exhale.

5. To finish, inhale deeply, and hold. Press your earlobe as hard as you can for a few seconds, and then exhale. Repeat twice.

TIPS

Moisten your lips to facilitate the whistling sound. You may feel some pain or discomfort at the beginning due to the loud sound in your head. Unless that feeling becomes painful, continue with the exercise.

PRECAUTIONS

Consult with your physician before performing it if you have brain tumors, epilepsy, or any brain-related conditions.

MEDITATION

This is a powerful reset that also brings instantaneous mindful alert. Imagine deleting (at least temporarily) all traumas, worries, and overthinking with this breathwork.

APPLICATIONS

- Sleep, rest, and vitality

- Holistic balance

- Neuroendocrine and metabolic regulation

28-DAY SOMATIC EVOLUTION CHALLENGE

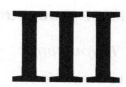

III

"I believe that discipline and self-love are the total secrets to freedom."
Anne Lamott

Freedom exists in being yourself and living with purpose, happiness, and well-being. Unhelpful habits, conditioning, and trauma can restrict our sense of freedom. That is why being free requires a kind of self-love related to daily practice, care, and commitment. And a crucial way to develop this mature self-love is to establish habits, like the somatic practices in this book, that allow you to confront what you consider authentically good for you and about you on a daily basis.

When you establish a habit, you open a space in your life to counteract and replace unconscious patterns with better ones. And this positive change will take hold on a subconscious level, sealing its effects long after the challenge is over. It can bring physical relief, increase your ability to cope with stressful situations, and foster healthier habits in your daily life.

This challenge invites you to commit to addressing the problems you need to resolve. You can use the structure of the challenge to build your own plan and consciously explore the somatic principles and practices that can target your individual wellness needs.

KEEP A JOURNAL

"If you cannot measure it, you cannot improve it."

William Kelvin

No matter how committed and inspired you are, it doesn't hurt to keep track of your routines. Use a journal to make notes on your progress during the 28-day challenge. Although digital notebooks work, it can be therapeutic to write by hand. Set aside a few minutes each day to reflect on your practice. If you can spend a few minutes to check-in with how you are feeling, what is helping, and what your intentions are for the week ahead, you may begin to observe subtle day-to-day changes and become more aware of the habits that help you stay on track over time.

DAILY REFLECTION

1. What do I need today?

2. Which somatic practices felt helpful?

3. Did anything (positively or negatively) impact my somatic practice?

4. How are the somatic exercises impacting my sense of well-being throughout the day?

5. Do I have any insights about something that has been causing discomfort or uneasiness?

WEEKLY REFLECTION

1. How am I feeling in the present moment?

2. What has changed? What have I learned to love and integrate this week?

3. What practices are helping (exercises, breathwork, meditation, diet, affirmations)?

4. What do I need to change or improve?

5. What aspect of my health will I focus on in the coming week?

28-DAY SOMATIC EVOLUTION PLAN

At the start of your 28-day challenge, it is beneficial to dedicate time to reflect on your most sincere intention for the weeks ahead. What do you want to change during this time? Define it well. Use deep breathing and mindful awareness to facilitate this process.

Identify (and write down) the benefits of fully committing yourself to completing the 28-day challenge. Evaluate the best time to perform the exercises each day, as well as all potential interruptions that may get in the way of your daily practice. Consider any aspects of your lifestyle that need to change in order to get the best results from your practices. It's best not to make too many changes at once so that you can focus your energy on your main goals.

Finally, set up a comfortable place where you can practice. Be sure to keep a yoga mat and cushion nearby.

TIPS

- Wait at least one hour after your last meal to perform any exercise, no matter how low-impact (except in the case of exercises suggested to improve digestion).

- Drink plenty of water when you practice.

- Perform the exercises slowly, and focus on body awareness and sensation.

- Explore the introductory exercises and resources. As you are just starting out, they will be very useful to help you have a better connection during the practice.

- Allow yourself to make adjustments to the content and order of your practice during this week as you get to know what works best for you.

- Get to know your stress responses and identify the energetic or emotional flooding you feel with the various exercises. It is important to get used to the idea of perceiving these flows and thus overcome the fear of emotional release.

- If you are short on time, you can choose to do an "express practice" instead of a full practice. In that case, slowly and mindfully perform three exercises from the indicated series, so that you still receive the somatic benefits each day.

WEEK ONE: PRACTICE BASIC SELF-REGULATION

To start the process, this week should be used to begin practicing the basics of self-regulation. These are usually the most difficult days to establish the habit, although you will certainly have the initial spark of motivation on your side.

	MONDAY	TUESDAY	WEDNESDAY	THURSDAY	FRIDAY	SATURDAY	SUNDAY
Complete Practice	Set I: Self-regulation, calmness, & rest	Set I: Self-regulation, calmness, & rest	Set I: Self-regulation, calmness, & rest	Set V: Self-love & emotional awareness	Set V: Self-love & emotional awareness	Set V: Self-love & emotional awareness	Rest and reflect in your journal
Or: Express Practice (less than 10 mins)	Exercises: 1, 3, 5	Exercises: 2, 4	Exercises: 1, 4, 6	Exercises: 25, 26, 30	Exercises: 25, 27, 29	Exercises: 26, 27, 28	

WEEK TWO: IDENTIFY WHAT NEEDS CHANGING

Now it is time to focus on what you consider to be your most significant needs. Identify which exercises could benefit you the most at this time, and integrate them into your practice this week.

	MONDAY	TUESDAY	WEDNESDAY	THURSDAY	FRIDAY	SATURDAY	SUNDAY
Complete Practice	Set II: Sleep, restoration, & vitality	Set III: Grounding & sciatic nerve health	Set III: Grounding & sciatic nerve health	Set IV: Spinal health & flexibility	Set IV: Spinal health & flexibility	Set II: Sleep, restoration, & vitality	Rest and reflect in your journal
Or: Express Practice (less than 10 mins)	Exercises: 7, 8, 9	Exercises: 13, 14, 17	Exercises: 15, 16, 18	Exercises: 19, 20, 24	Exercises: 21, 22, 23	Sleep set: 10, 11, 12	
Plus one additional daily exercise	Choose at least one Stage II exercise to address your most significant needs, and integrate this into your daily practice for the entire length of the challenge.						

WEEK THREE: DEEPEN THE SOMATIC PRACTICE

By now you have become familiar with your main exercise, and have accumulated sufficient expertise about the execution of somatic exercises. Considering that you have already improved your ability to self-regulate at least at a basic level, it's time to deepen your health and harmony using resources from Stage 2 while still focusing on your main issue through your daily exercise.

	MONDAY	TUESDAY	WEDNESDAY	THURSDAY	FRIDAY	SATURDAY	SUNDAY
Complete Practice	Stage 2 Set I: Vagus nerve regulation	Stage 2 Set I: Vagus nerve regulation	Stage 2 Set I: Vagus nerve regulation	Stage 2 Set II: Neuroendocrine & metabolic regulation	Stage 2 Set III: Pleasure, joy, and sexual health	Stage 2 Set II: Neuroendocrine & metabolic regulation	Rest and reflect in your journal
Or: Express Practice (less than 10 mins)	Exercises: 31, 32, 35	Exercises: 31, 32, 35	Exercises: 32, 33, 34	Exercises: 36, 38, 40	Exercises: 41, 45	Exercises: 37, 38, 40	
Plus one additional daily exercise	Choose a set of your choice to practice this week. Consider choosing the same set as the one your daily exercise is in so that you can work on the issue in a more comprehensive way.						

WEEK FOUR: INTEGRATE WHAT YOU HAVE LEARNED

You have gotten to know yourself pretty well and have become accustomed to the routine. Use your resources to stay present and actively engaged. Try to use sets that favor integration so that you consolidate what you have learned.

	MONDAY	TUESDAY	WEDNESDAY	THURSDAY	FRIDAY	SATURDAY	SUNDAY
Complete Practice	Stage 2 Set III: Pleasure, joy, and sexual health	Stage 2 Set II: Neuroendocrine & metabolic regulation	Stage 2 Set IV: Holistic balance	Stage 2 Set IV: Holistic balance	Stage 2 Set V: Mindful alert & focus	Stage 2 Set V: Mindful alert & focus	Celebrate, rest, and reflect.
Or: Express Practice (less than 10 mins)	Exercises: 43, 42, 44	Exercises: 37, 39, 40	Exercises: 46, 47, 48, 49	Exercises: 46, 47, 48, 50	Exercises: 51, 52, 53, 55	Exercises: 51, 52, 54, 55	
Plus one additional daily exercise	Consider incorporating one of the more spontaneous introductory exercises like "Shake it off" or "Dance."						

CLOSURE AND REST

It is very useful to dedicate at least one day to reflect on the process of transformation, and take time to feel gratitude and celebrate. After completing the 28-day challenge, you can repeat the challenge, and vary the sets to fit your particular needs.

ESTABLISH HEALTHY HABITS

There are many suggestions for a healthy lifestyle. However, there are some common patterns that can be integrated to promote embodiment.

HYDRATION

It is best to hydrate with plain water. Listen to your body and drink when you feel thirsty. Try to get in the habit of drinking water before going to sleep, and upon waking up.

NOURISHMENT

Try to eat natural food instead of processed food as much as possible, and choose food that has been prepared healthfully (for instance steamed, boiled, grilled, stewed, or fermented). Consuming plenty of complex carbohydrates (fruits and tubers), instead of simple and refined carbohydrates (such as flour) will help regulate blood glucose, improve energy, and regulate your ability to focus and concentrate. Choose natural sweeteners (honey and cane sugar) and sea salt whenever possible.

Your metabolism can benefit from a healthy eating rhythm, with at least four hours for your digestion to rest between meals. Likewise, if you can avoid carbohydrates at dinner time, and finish eating early it can improve your sleep and help you wake up with more energy. For some people, intermittent fasting for 12 to 16 hours a few times a week can be very beneficial. If you are interested in intermittent fasting, consult a dietician to learn about the different ways you can create a fasting schedule that works for your particular body and needs. (Intermittent fasting is not recommended if you have a history of disordered eating).

Eat slowly to promote better digestion and weight control. Try to use meal times to practice awareness through your senses of taste and smell, and listen to your body's signals to let you know when you feel full.

SLEEP

Good sleep is an essential part of health and well-being. To establish good sleep habits, it is recommended that you try to get at least seven to eight hours of sleep each night, and regularly go to bed early. In the hour before bed, try to dim the lights and avoid devices, as well as any other sources of overstimulation or stress. Take time to talk with those close to you and do restorative activities like taking a bath, meditating, stretching, or journaling.

POSTURE, BODY, AND MOVEMENT

If you take the time to improve your posture, flexibility, and alignment, it can benefit your overall well-being. Spend at least 20 minutes a day stretching and exercising. Make a habit of maintaining good upright posture. When standing, especially for long periods of time, try to center your weight on the metatarsus (the central segment of the foot) and not on the heel, which can cause compression in the lumbar area.

When sitting at your desk, avoid slouching and take regular breaks to stretch, take a walk, and massage your shoulders and neck. Take care of ergonomics in the different spaces in your life. For example: sit in a comfortable chair when working, adjust the monitor, keyboard and mouse to the ideal height, and feel comfortable when driving.

ENVIRONMENT AND SURROUNDINGS

Spend time in nature as much as possible. Notice the beauty of the details around you. Take time to walk outside, walk barefoot, sunbathe, and swim. Wherever you are, take time to pay attention to the natural elements like the weather, the temperature, the ground beneath your feet, and the sounds like birds, wind, or water.

Maintain a clean and orderly environment both at work and at home. Personalize your space so that it feels calm and grounding. Use natural aromas, lighting, colors, and plants that make the environment feel peaceful. Consider reducing your exposure to Wi-Fi and phone signals as much as possible to reduce inflammatory responses and distraction.

REST AND REPLENISH

Take time to regularly rest and replenish your inner resources with creative activities. For instance, try singing, dancing, playing music, making art, or cooking. Creative activities, play, and laughter can have significant therapeutic benefits, like reducing stress, fostering a sense of embodiment, self-awareness, and connection.

REFERENCES

[1]Shapiro, L. (2020). The Somatic Therapy Workbook: Stress-Relieving Exercises for Strengthening the Mind-Body Connection and Sparking Emotional and Physical Healing.

[2]Hanna, T. "What is Somatics?" Retrieved from URL: https://somatics.org/library/htl-wis1

[3]Tougaw, J. (2019). "What is Somatics?" Retrieved from URL: https://www.psychologytoday.com/us/blog/the-elusive-brain/201904/what-is-somatics

[4]Nijenhuis, E. R. S. "Somatoform Dissociation: Major Symptoms of Dissociative Disorders." Journal of Trauma & Dissociation. 1.4 (2001): 7–32. https://doi.org/10.1300/J229v01n04_02

[5]Nummenmaa, L., and H. Saarimäki. "Emotions as Discrete Patterns of Systemic Activity." Neuroscience Letters. 693 (2019): 3–8. https://doi.org/10.1016/j.neulet.2017.07.012

[6]Vendrell, I. "Emotions and Sentiments: Two Distinct Forms of Affective Intentionality." Phenomenology and Mind. 23 (2022): 20–34.

[7]Skylight (2023). "What is Spiritual Stress?" Retrieved from URL: https://skylight.org/blog/posts/what-is-spiritual-distress

[8]Porges, Stephen. "Vagal Tone: A Physiologic Marker of Stress Vulnerability." Pediatrics. 90 (1992): 498–504. 10.1542/peds.90.3.498.

[9]Charles, S. T., et al. "The Wear and Tear of Daily Stressors on Mental Health." Psychological Science, 24.5 (2013): 733–741. https://doi.org/10.1177/0956797612462222

[10]Vaskovic, J. (2023). Nervous System. Retrieved from URL: https://www.kenhub.com/en/library/anatomy/the-nervous-system

[11]Trivedi, Gunjan Y, et al. "Effect of Lifestyle Choices on Cerebrospinal Fluid Pulsations." Journal of Applied Consciousness Studies. 12.1 (Jan-June 2024): 58–64. DOI: 10.4103/jacs.jacs_42_23

[12]Gershon M. D. "The Enteric Nervous System: A Second Brain." Hospital Practice. 34.7 (1995). https://doi.org/10.3810/hp.1999.07.153

[13]Mischke-Reeds, M. (2018). Somatic Psychotherapy Toolbox: 125 Worksheets and Exercises to Treat Trauma & Stress. Retrieved from https://www.amazon.co.uk/Somatic-Psychotherapy-Toolbox-Worksheets-Exercises/dp/1683731352

[14]Snape, J. (2024). "The Power of Proprioception: How to Improve Your 'Sixth Sense'—and Become Healthier and Happier." Retrieved from: https://www.theguardian.com/lifeandstyle/article/2024/jul/18/the-power-of-proprioception-how-to-improve-your-sixth-sense-and-become-healthier-and-happier

[15]Baxter, R. (2023). "Organs of the eEndocrine System." Retrieved from URL: https://www.kenhub.com/en/library/anatomy/endocrine-system

[15]Homo Medicus (2024). "Cuáles son las Funciones Endocrinas del Hígado." Retrieved from URL: https://homomedicus.com/cuales-son-las-funciones-endocrinas-del-higado/

[16]Shahid, S. (2023). Thymus. Retrieved from URL: https://www.kenhub.com/en/library/anatomy/thymus

[17]Telles, S., and N. Singh. "'Science of the Mind: Ancient Yoga Texts and Modern Studies." The Psychiatric Clinics of North America. 36.1 (2013): 93–108. https://doi.org/10.1016/j.psc.2013.01.010

[18]Brown, R. P., and P.L. Gerbarg. "Yoga Breathing, Meditation, and Longevity." Annals of the New York Academy of Sciences. 1172 (2009): 54–62. https://doi.org/10.1111/j.1749-6632.2009.04394.x

[19]Nairn, R. (2022). "Timing is Everything: Why Eating on a Regular Schedule Supports Overall Well-Being." Retrieved from URL: https://wellbeing.jhu.edu/blog/2022/12/09/timing-is-everything-why-eating-on-a-regular-schedule-supports-overall-well-being/

[20]Manzella, D. (2024). Understanding Simple and Complex Carbohydrates. Retrieved from URL: https://www.verywellhealth.com/simple-and-complex-carbohydrates-1087570

[21]Hawton, K., et al. "Slow Down: Behavioral and Physiological Effects of Reducing Eating Rate." Nutrients. 11 (2019): 50. https://doi.org/10.3390/nu11010050

[22]Blume, C., et al. "Effects of Light on Human Circadian Rhythms, Sleep and Mood." Somnologie : Schlafforschung und Schlafmedizin Somnology: Sleep Research and Sleep Medicine, 23.3 (2019): 147–156. https://doi.org/10.1007/s11818-019-00215-x

[23]Pall M. L. "Wi-Fi is an Important Threat to Human Health." Environmental Research. 164 (2018): 405–416. https://doi.org/10.1016/j.envres.2018.01.035

[24]Hamel, J. (2021). Somatic Therapy: Alleviating Pain and Trauma through Art. Retrieved from: https://www.amazon.com/Somatic-Art-Therapy-Alleviating-through/dp/0367903237

BONUS THANK YOU

Thank you for choosing **Somatic Exercises for Nervous System Regulation 101**. We hope this book has provided you with the guidance and inspiration needed for your wellness journey. Your commitment to improving your health and well-being is truly commendable. Remember, every small step you take brings you closer to a healthier, happier you. Keep going, and stay motivated!

Don't forget to claim your bonus. Go to your internet browser and type in **https://www.getmovefit.com/somaticexercises** to register for the unlimited and free portal access. There are no hidden extra costs, this is completely free with the purchase of this book.

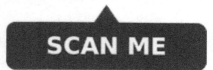

THE PIN CODE TO
UNLOCK YOUR BONUS IS

22566

WE ARE HERE TO HELP! Contact us at **support@getmovefit.com** and we will reply within 2 business days.

These bonuses are **FREE** and designed to **help you achieve your goals**.

With gratitude,
Linette Cunley

Made in United States
Orlando, FL
29 November 2024